PRACTICAL STATISTICS
for the HEALTH SCIENCES

Peter **MARTIN** • Robyn **PIERCE**
The University of Ballarat

Nelson

An International Thomson Publishing Company

Melbourne • Bonn • Boston • London • Madrid • Mexico City • New York • Paris • Singapore
Tokyo • Toronto • Albany NY • Belmont CA • Cincinnati OH • Detroit MI

Thomas Nelson Australia
102 Dodds Street
South Melbourne 3205

I(T)P Thomas Nelson Australia is an International Thomson
Publishing company

First published 1994
10 9 8 7 6 5 4 3 2 1
99 98 97 96 95 94

National Library of Australia
Cataloguing-in-Publication data

Martin, Peter, 1949– .
   Practical statistics for the health sciences.
   Includes index.
   ISBN 0 17 008976 2.
   1. Medical statistics. I. Pierce, Robyn, 1952– . II. Title.
519.502461

Designed by Erika Budiman
Cover designed by Erika Budiman
Cover illustration by Michelle Ryan
Typeset by Eclipse Graphics
Printed in Australia by McPherson's Printing Group

Nelson Australia Pty Limited ACN 004 603 454 (incorporated in
Victoria) trading as Thomas Nelson Australia.

The I(T)P trademark is used under licence.

Within the publishing process Thomas Nelson Australia uses resources,
technology and suppliers that are as environmentally friendly as
possible.

Contents

Change rocks nurses' boat

Much of what now seems basic in modern health care can be traced to pitched battles fought by Florence Nightingale in the 19th century. Less well known, because it has been neglected by her biographers, is her equally pioneering use of the new advanced techniques of statistical analysis in those battles. ...in addition to advancing the cause of medical reform itself she helped to pioneer the revolutionary notion that social phenomena could be objectively measured and subjected to mathematical analysis.

PREFACE

This quotation was taken from an article by I. Bernard Cohen in *Scientific American* (volume 250, issue 3, March 1984). The article went on to emphasise the important role played by Florence Nightingale in the saving of thousands of lives of soldiers in the Crimean War. Her use of statistics to show that the main cause of death in war was disease rather than wounds sustained in battle still speaks eloquently today. She effectively demonstrated that statistics provide an organised way of learning from experience and could lead to improvement in medical and surgical practice.

Today basic nursing education is not only about preparing nurses to work in hospitals, but also in independent practice, health promotion and community health centres. With this increasing professionalism comes a greater need for critical thinkers, particularly in the light of current technological advances. Modern technological developments and advances in our knowledge in general emphasise more than ever the need for an understanding of the general aspects of statistical analysis.

In most fields of human endeavour, there is at one time or another a need to collect and examine data; that is, information in numerical or quantitative form. A well-educated person in any field should have an appreciation of the basic ideas involved in collecting, presenting, and analysing data. A knowledge of statistics is essential for those who wish to evaluate or become involved in any kind of research. It can be useful in deciding on the validity of claims made by others, or in the design and conduct of investigations. A basic understanding of statistics can be an invaluable asset when communicating with professional colleagues, particularly in the effective presentation of findings resulting from research.

With increasing professionalism, nurses need to keep abreast of developments in their field, which are usually written up in scientific journals. It is important for the professional nurse to have the necessary skills to read these journals and to be able to review and understand them.

The material in this text has been developed over a number of years, during which we have been involved in teaching service courses in statistics to nursing students. We have found that students in this field wish to relate their learning to their chosen vocation, so we have familiarised ourselves with current nursing research and developed teaching examples accordingly.

Course outlines

The following flow charts provide suggested course outlines for one-semester courses in basic descriptive statistics and statistical inference. If a two-semester course is required, these charts placed end-to-end would provide the basis for a fully comprehensive course in introductory statistics.

Chart 1: One-semester course in basic descriptive statistics

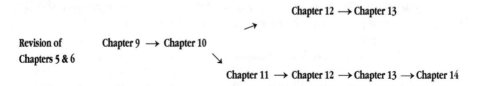

Chart 2: One-semester course in statistical inference

Chapter 12 → Chapter 13

Revision of   Chapter 9 → Chapter 10
Chapters 5 & 6

Chapter 11 → Chapter 12 → Chapter 13 → Chapter 14

We would like to acknowledge, with thanks, the support we have received from our respective children, James and Michael, and Kari and Anna, for the time we have not been able to spend with them during the writing of this book. Special thanks to Peter's wife Pauline for her practical help and support, and to Robyn's husband David for his assistance, particularly the out-of-hours medical consultations regarding birth weights, breast feeding, disease data, and so on.

Also, we would especially like to acknowledge the assistance and support we have received from Lyn Roberts (School of Mathematics and Computing, University of Ballarat). Her critical comments and suggestions have been greatly appreciated and have helped us to bridge the gap between theory and practice.

CHAPTER OUTLINE

1.1 Definitions
Definitions and explanations of key words used in statistics.

1.2 Number scales
Different types of data and the scales used for measurement.

1.3 Discrete and continuous variables
The distinction between discrete and continuous variables.

1.4 Summary: the first important steps
Applying the chapter contents to statistical problems.

CHAPTER ONE

Basic terms and number scales

After studying this chapter you should be able to:

- identify the key elements of a real-world problem that could be solved using statistics;
- start using statistical terms correctly;
- distinguish different types of data and know the limitations of the mathematics that is appropriate to use with each type; and
- recognise discrete and continuous variables.

Taking a person's blood pressure involves following certain procedures in order to obtain a result which can then be analysed. Obtaining an accurate temperature reading or pulse rate for a patient also involves following certain procedures to obtain a satisfactory result. Statistics is a bit similar in that it is a collection of techniques and procedures that assist the researcher to organise and summarise data. These techniques allow us to make inferences about the data and to effectively communicate the results to others. In order to make full use of statistical procedures we need to be able to speak its language, and we need to define some basic terms. The following definitions are descriptive in nature; they are not meant to be mathematically complete.

1.1   Definitions

Population

A population consists of the complete set or group of individuals, objects, or scores that the investigator is interested in studying. Populations may be very large or they may be quite narrowly defined. For example, a social worker studying the effects of unemployment may define the population as those people unemployed in Australia or, more narrowly, as those unemployed in a particular city or town.

Sample

The sample is a *subset of the population*. In many experimental situations researchers collect data from samples that have been selected from defined populations. Collecting information from samples usually costs less, takes less time, and (providing the sample has been properly selected) can give an accurate reflection of the population at large. The art of statistical research and analysis is to be able to *generalise* from the sample to the population with some degree of confidence.

Variables and constants

A variable is some characteristic or property of some event, object, or person that can take different values at different times, depending on the conditions. Height, weight, reaction time and drug dosage are examples of variables. A variable should be contrasted with a constant, which, of course, does not have different values at different times. An example of a constant is the number of millilitres in a litre. This always has the same value (1000 mL = 1 litre).

Control variable (independent variable)

The control variable in an experiment is the variable that is *systematically manipulated* by the investigator. In most experiments the investigator is interested in determining the effect that one variable may have on one or more other variables. For example, suppose you are interested in the effects of alcohol on reaction time.

By varying the amount of alcohol present in the bloodstreams of the subjects, you can investigate the effects upon reaction time. In this case the amount of alcohol in the bloodstream is the control variable because its levels are controlled by the experimenter, independent of any change in the other variables. In this example, you are manipulating the amount of alcohol and measuring the effect on reaction time. Alcohol amount is the control variable.

In another experiment, the effect of sleep deprivation on aggressive behaviour may be studied. Subjects are deprived of various amounts of sleep, and the effect on aggressiveness is observed. Here, the amount of sleep deprivation is the variable being manipulated, so it is the control variable. When the results are plotted on a graph, the control variable is usually put on the horizontal axis.

Dependent (response) variable

The dependent (or response) variable in an experiment is the variable that is affected by the control variable. A researcher measures the dependent variable in order to determine the effect of the control variable. For example, in the experiment studying the effects of alcohol on reaction time, the reaction times of the subjects are measured to see if they are affected by the amount of alcohol consumed. Thus, reaction time is the dependent variable. It is called 'dependent' because it may depend on the amount of alcohol consumed.

In the investigation of sleep deprivation and aggressive behaviour, the amount of sleep deprivation is being manipulated, and the aggressive behaviour of the subjects is being measured. Amount of sleep deprivation is the independent variable and aggressive behaviour is the dependent variable.

Data

Data forms the raw material for statistical analysis. A data value is simply a piece of information that may be numerical (for example, a patient's temperature) or nonnumerical (a patient's blood type). Any measurements that are made on a particular variable are called data. Data may consist of measurements of characteristics, such as age, sex, number of beds available, etc. Numerical data values, as originally measured, are often referred to as *raw* or *original scores*. Alternatively, data may consist of the responses to a particular survey which may or may not involve numerical quantities.

Statistic

A statistic is a number calculated from the *sample data*. It quantifies some characteristic of the sample we might be interested in exploring, such as centre or spread. Examples of such statistics are *averages, standard deviations, correlation coefficients*.

Parameter

A parameter is a number calculated from *population data*. It quantifies a characteristic of the population. For example, the average value of a population set of scores is called a parameter, whereas the average value of a sample of scores is called a statistic. Statistics and parameters are very similar concepts. Statistics are based upon samples, and their values vary depending upon the sample chosen. Parameters, on the other hand, are defined with respect to their particular populations.

EXAMPLE 1.1

For the following experimental case, identify the population, the sample, the independent variable, the dependent variable, the data and the statistics.

A clinical nurse teacher believes that different methods of teaching will produce different results from her students. A group of 50 first-year nursing students is selected from all the first-year nurses at a particular institution to participate in an experiment designed to test the teacher's belief. Half the students are taught using conventional teaching methods, while the remaining half are taught using a new method devised by the teacher. At the end of the semester the 50 students sit for the same exam. The average score for both groups is calculated and compared to see if there is any difference.

The *population* is all first-year student nurses enrolled at the particular institution.

The *sample* is the 50 first-year students selected to participate in the experiment.

The *independent variable* is the method of teaching used.

The *dependent variable* is student performance in the examination.

The *data* is the examination scores of the 50 students.

The *statistics* are the average scores for both groups.

1.2 Number scales

In order for a student to travel the 7 kilometres from her home to university she must catch the number 42 bus. Her bus fare costs $1.50 and crosses 3 fare zones. The numbers in this statement are being used in quite different ways, and without thinking we naturally treat them differently. It doesn't take very much to realise that bus number 42 is not twice as fast (or twice as anything for that matter) as bus number 21. The number 42 simply identifies the route that a particular bus takes. Three fare zones is further than one fare zone, but it is not necessarily three times as far because each zone may be a different distance. However, we can say that 7 kilometres is twice as far as 3.5 kilometres and $1.50 is three times as much as 50 cents, or half as much as $3.00. We intuitively treat these numbers differently because *they involve different levels*, or *scales*, *of measurement*.

From the above example we see that numbers may be used for a variety of purposes. They may be used as labels, or to indicate rank, or to represent actual quantities. It is these three uses of numbers that are of particular interest to us. Not recognising the purpose for which a set of numbers is being used can easily cause confusion; worse still, it can lead to the calculation of quite meaningless statistics. For example, in order for a nursing student to travel from home to the hospital where she has been placed for clinicals, she must catch the number 42 bus into the city, then the number 9 bus to the sporting complex, and finally the number 12 bus to get to the hospital. The average of these numbers is 21, but what meaning does this average convey? In the context of the example this statistic is meaningless, because the numbers are being used as labels. That is, they are only being used to identify particular routes that the various buses take throughout the city. While it is possible to calculate an average, the purpose for which the numbers are being used renders the calculation meaningless.

Applying numbers to concepts in accordance with some set of rules is known as scaling. When creating scales we use as much appropriate information as is available and measure as accurately as the measuring instrument will allow.

Using numbers as labels

When numbers are used as labelling devices we cannot use them in calculations as we would in normal arithmetic; all we can meaningfully do is count the frequency of similar objects. Using numbers in this way is referred to as using a *nominal scale of measurement*, which really amounts to classifying the objects and giving them a number to identify the name of the category to which they belong. For example, most tertiary institutions use numbers to identify students; every driver has a licence number; hospitals use ward numbers to designate particular wards; and athletes and football players have identifying numbers as labels.

While numbers used in this way are referred to as a nominal scale, they do not really form a scale at all: they are simply numbers being used to represent categories for identification purposes. There is no suggestion of using these kinds of numbers for true measurements, because they are being used to represent what we call *categorical* or *qualitative* data. Our primary interest with such data is to determine which of the categories occurs most (or least) often. The coding of categories using numbers is particularly useful in computer analysis of the data. For example, Males = 1, Females = 0.

Ordinal data: using numbers as ranks

Salary scales are examples of using numbers as *ranks*. A person on a Level 1 salary scale may receive an annual salary of $25,450. A Level 2 salary might be $27,900 per year, while a Level 3 salary might be $30,050. Note that these salary levels may only apply to a particular workplace. Similarly, the order in which a list of jobs is to be completed may well be ranked according to particular priorities. The order in which athletes finish a race is another example of numbers being used as rankings.

In these instances the people or objects being measured are ranked in order, so the scale is called an *ordinal scale*. The *order* is defined according to whether they possess more (or less) of the variable that is being measured. Ranking consists of arranging a number of objects so that each object is greater (or more intense with respect to some particular characteristic) than the one placed next to it. Some form of ranking is almost always used in sport as a measure of performance. While we can say that the player ranked 1st is *better* than the player ranked 2nd, who in turn is *better* than the player ranked 3rd, we cannot say that the player ranked 1st is twice as good as the player ranked 2nd. Nor can we say that the difference between the 1st and the 2nd rankings is the same as the difference between the 2nd and the 3rd rankings.

Ranking scales such as those just mentioned tell us nothing about the magnitude of the difference between adjacent units, nor do they have the property of equal intervals between adjacent units. All we can say is that one particular player is better than some other player, or that some *thing* possesses more (or less) of a certain attribute than another thing. Differences between the times of two runners, for example, indicate how far apart they finished in a particular race, whereas the differences in their placings do not. Ordinal scales do not specify the distance between any of the given categories. If only ordinal data is available, we can say that a patient is more satisfied than another patient, but we cannot say that one patient is twice as satisfied as another.

Metric scales of measurement

Measurement scales in which the distances between any two numbers on the scale are of known and equal size are often called *metric scales of measurement*. For example, if one patient has a temperature of 38°C and another has a temperature of 42°C then we know that the first patient has a temperature that is 4° *higher* than the second patient. If one patient weighs 45 kg and another weighs 90 kg we can also say that the first patient weighs only half as much as the second. These examples of metric scales of measurement produce more refined distinctions in the measurement process than ordinal scales or ranking scales. In fact, the two examples of metric scales used here highlight the two important categories that arise within this measurement scale. Metric scales of measurement consist of *interval-measuring scales* or *ratio-measuring scales*.

Interval scales of measurement

The Celsius and Fahrenheit temperature scales are good examples of interval scales of measurement. The additional heat indicated by a change in temperature from 5° to 6° is the same as that indicated by a change in temperature from 100° to 101°. Equal amounts of heat are indicated between adjacent units throughout the scale.

A characteristic of such scales of measurement is that the value *zero* does not represent the *absolute* zero point; that is, the total absence of whatever it is that is being measured. Zero on the Celsius scale for example is only an arbitrary zero point that happens to be the temperature at which water freezes. On the Fahrenheit scale the same amount of heat is indicated by a value of 32°.

Operating mathematically with such a scale is limited to adding and subtracting. For example, if today's maximum temperature was 20°C and tomorrow is forecast to be 5° warmer, then we can look forward to a maximum of 25°C tomorrow. What we cannot say, however, is that a temperature of 20°C is twice as hot as 10°C.

Ratio scales of measurement

Ratio scales represent the highest level of measurement and are used for measuring variables such as height, weight, distance, frequencies of events, time, etc. In addition to all of the properties of interval scales, ratio scales have an absolute zero point. This allows us to calculate ratios and perform all the other mathematical operations that usually are associated with numbers. With ratio scales we are able to say that a particular object is twice as heavy as another, or that it took me only half the time to complete a task as it took somebody else.

Test scales

Most of us at some time or another have taken part in a test or an examination. Teachers and behavioural scientists use tests as tools to measure a variety of variables — knowledge of a particular subject, IQ, anxiety, attitude, and so forth. In the light of the above discussion, what measuring scale is being used when we score students on a test of Mathematics or English Literature? Do such variables have an absolute zero point? Can we be sure that such variables possess equal intervals between adjacent units? Questions like these need to be thought about before drawing conclusions based upon the results achieved, or not achieved, when using test scales of measurement. If there is a choice of scales available then we should use the scale which allows us to record the most information.

1.3   *Discrete and continuous variables*

It is important to know the type of variable that is being studied, because this will influence the statistical analysis applied. In a broad sense variables are classified as either *qualitative* or *quantitative*. Blood types, sex, racial origin, and cause of death are qualitative variables, for which a nominal scale of measurement is used. Quantitative variables are measured using either ordinal or metric scales of measurement. Furthermore, quantitative variables that are measured using metric scales can be further categorised as being *discrete* or *continuous*.

Variables such as the number of children in a family, the number of heartbeats in a given time period, the number of live births last month, the sum of two dice in a game of Monopoly, or the number of imported cars sold in this country last year, are examples of *discrete* variables. These are variables that are usually analysed by counting the number of individuals, or items, that fall into specified categories. *Continuous* variables, on the other hand can theoretically assume an infinite number of possible values between any two adjacent points on the scale, and are usually *measured* rather than counted. Examples of continuous variables include height, weight, time, distance, blood pressure, age, temperature, and so on.

1.4 Summary: the first important steps

When confronted with a body of data for analysis there are three important initial steps for organising the way in which you think about data:

(a) observe how many variables are present,

(b) determine what type of variables are present, and

(c) establish which measuring scale is being used for each variable.

Having done this you will be in a position to organise the raw data into meaningful displays using appropriate tables and graphs, or to calculate representative statistics.

1 A community health nurse was planning a course in effective parenting for the people in his area. In preparation for this he obtained information about the entire city from the Bureau of Statistics and collected data from a sample of families residing in the suburbs where he worked. The results obtained appear below.

Number of children per family	Number of families (in city)	Number of families (in the sample)
0	120	6
1	180	10
2	270	12
3	300	8
4	80	6
5	50	8

(a) Identify the elements of the population and give the population size.

(b) Identify the elements of the sample and give the sample size.

(c) Suppose the nurse was interested in the number of families with more than two children. What are the values of the statistic and the parameter?

(d) Suppose the nurse was interested in the proportion of families with less than four children. What are the values of the statistic and the parameter?

2 Administrative personnel at a training hospital wanted to estimate the average admission time for the 550 patients currently in the hospital. Statistically minded secretarial staff selected an initial sample of 10 patients in order to make their estimate. The average admission time for the sample was 45 minutes.

(a) What is the population, and how many data values does it contain?

(b) What is the parameter of interest?

(c) What is the value of the statistic that is used to estimate the parameter?

(d) Suppose another sample of 10 patients was selected. Would it be likely that the value of the statistic is the same as that from the initial sample? Why? Would the value of the parameter remain the same?

CHAPTER OUTLINE

2.1 Frequency tables
The importance of organising data and some guidelines for organisation.

2.2 Bar graphs and pie graphs
Illustrating data which is only scaled by categories.

2.3 Histograms and frequency polygons
Illustrating data which has metric scaling.

2.4 Line graphs
Construction and application of line graphs; constructing cumulative frequency polygons.

2.5 Percentile points and percentile ranks
Using ogives to find key values in a distribution.

2.6 Stem-and-leaf displays
A method of organising and displaying data without losing any detail.

2.7 The pros and cons of grouping data
A summary of the arguments for and against grouping data.

2.8 Minitab
An introduction to the Minitab statistical software; using Minitab to display data.

CHAPTER TWO

Displaying raw data

After studying this chapter you should be able to:
- construct a frequency table using suitable interval bounds;
- choose an appropriate statistical graph to display data;
- draw clearly labelled statistical graphs;
- interpret data from statistical graphs;
- calculate percentile points and percentile ranks from an ogive;
- construct a stem-and-leaf display; and
- use Minitab to enter and graph data.

If a picture is worth a thousand words then a good graph is worth a thousand numbers. When dealing with numerical information the use of visual communication is even more important, because while most people would read 1000 words if necessary, few would bother to look at 1000 numbers. So graphs are used to:

- simplify information,
- communicate a message, and
- gain a reader's attention.

We see them in daily newspapers, professional journals, reports, and so forth. In many instances the main emphasis in these presentations of the data is to catch the eye of the reader, or to enable the reader to readily see the most important aspects of the data. Unfortunately, in some cases accuracy is overlooked in order to emphasise some particular point. An illustration of this can be seen in the following examples.

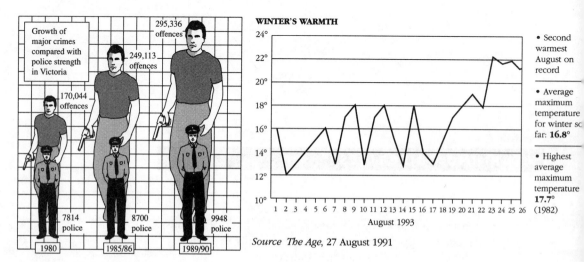

Source *Herald-Sun*, 11 June 1991, p5

Source *The Age*, 27 August 1991

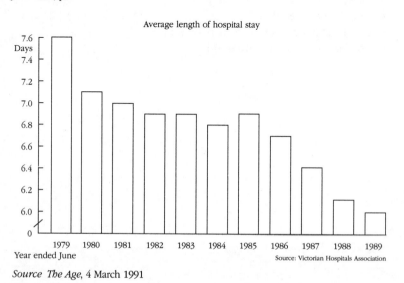

Source *The Age*, 4 March 1991

Figure 2.1 Emphasising a particular aspect of data in a graph can sometimes lead to visual distortion and misinterpretation.

Practical statistics for the health sciences

When it is important for the reader to know something of the actual numbers involved, and not just see a trend, or pattern, then raw data should be summarised in the form of a table. Data presented in its raw form does not communicate very well at all. This is because any underlying trends or patterns which may be present in the data are easily hidden amongst all of the detail. In its raw form data may consist of an unordered collection of observations, recorded in a note book or on a specific recording sheet, or even on a scrap of paper.

By presenting raw data in an orderly fashion we enable the important features of the data to be highlighted. This is more efficient and allows us to make comparisons with other data sets more easily. The main reason for organising raw data into tables and graphs is to see if there is any underlying structure in the data. How does a patient's temperature vary over a given period of time? Which form of health insurance is the most popular with younger people? Does the data have a particular shape when it is graphed? Where is the centre of the data, and how spread out is the data? These are the sorts of questions that we may wish to investigate in any initial *exploratory data analysis*. These characteristics can be further used in inferential analysis, as we shall see in later sections. Various forms of tables, graphs and pictographs may be used to display and organise data, depending upon the purpose of the investigator, and also on the nature of the data. Some of the more common methods of data presentation are discussed below.

2.1 Frequency tables

Often the first step in organising raw data is to arrange the data into some sort of tabular form. One of the simplest tables to construct is a *frequency table*. Such a table usually has *two* columns — one dealing with *categories,* or *intervals of values,* and the other dealing with *frequencies.* Frequency means the number of times that a particular value occurs in a set of data, or the number of times a particular category occurs.

In Example 2.1 the order of the blood types is not important in the sense that type A does not necessarily have to come before type B and so on. This is an example of a *nominal scale* of measurement. Note, however, that the blood types have been arranged in order in the table, according to their respective frequencies. The most common blood type has been listed first. This is often done in such tables because it is often the main point of interest.

EXAMPLE **2.1**

The blood types of 40 volunteer blood donors was collected with the following results. Arrange these results into a simple frequency table.

Raw Data: O O A B A O A A A O A A A B A A O O A AB
             B O B O O A O O A A O O A A A O A O O AB

Solution

Blood type	Frequency
A	18
O	16
B	4
AB	2
Total	40

The following graph taken from a local country newspaper has a different purpose. In this case the main emphasis is to inform the community of the current stocks of the local blood bank. Hopefully this will result in concerned blood donors donating the required blood types before stocks run out completely.

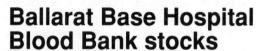

Ballarat Base Hospital Blood Bank stocks

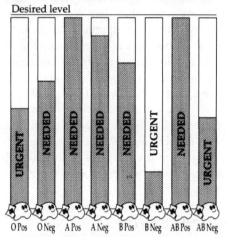

Desired level

O Pos   O Neg   A Pos   A Neg   B Pos   B Neg   AB Pos   AB Neg

Blood Bank hours: Monday 2pm to 8pm; Tuesday, Wednesday and Thursday, 2pm to 5pm; Friday, closed. Office opens 1pm daily, first floor, Base Hospital, phone (053) 204341.

Source: The Ballarat Courier

Figure 2.2 A bar graph that gets its important message across clearly and succinctly.

Example 2.2 shows a frequency table that is similar to that in Example 2.1, but this time the data has been measured using a *continuous scale*. In addition, this example uses intervals (ranges of values) of scores rather than individual categories, as was the case in Example 2.1. When using intervals in this manner, three points should be kept in mind:

1 Use interval widths that are easy to deal with.

2 Make sure that every score is included in *one* interval only.

3 Limit the number of intervals to between 5 and 20.

EXAMPLE	**2.2**

Arrange the following student examination scores into a suitable table.

Raw Scores
78 37 99 66 90 79 80 89 68 57 71 78 53 81 77 58 93
79 88 76 60 77 49 92 83 80 74 69 90 62 84 64 73 48
75 98 42 75 84 87 65 59 63 86 95 55 70 62 85 72

EXAMPLE 2.2   cont.

Solution

Score interval	Frequency
30 – 39	1
40 – 49	3
50 – 59	5
60 – 69	9
70 – 79	14
80 – 89	11
90 – 99	7
Total	50

The width chosen for intervals (sometimes called *class intervals*) is subjective to some extent. The wider the interval, the fewer intervals you have in the resulting table. Information is *lost* because the data is *compressed* into such intervals. This can lead to an unclear display of the shape of the distribution of the data. On the other hand, the narrower the interval, the more faithfully the original data are preserved. However, an interval that is too narrow will also lead to an unclear display of the shape of the distribution because the data will be spread too thinly over too many intervals (Figure 2.3).

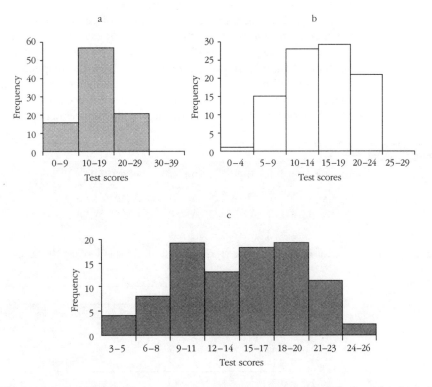

Figure 2.3 An interval that is too wide or too narrow leads to an unclear display of the shape of the distribution. In this example, (c) provides the best display of the distribution.

The three graphs have been prepared from the same set of data. In each case the score interval is different and the resulting effect on the shape of the graphs is obvious. The interval sizes are 10, 5 and 3 respectively. Graphs a and b have too few intervals, thereby compressing the data too much. The *bimodal* nature of the data (that is, the two-peaked appearance in graph c) is not evident until the interval width is reduced to 3. Other common interval sizes are 3, 5, 10, 20, 50, 100, etc. The size chosen should provide a meaningful visual display.

2.2 Bar graphs and pie graphs

Data can often be displayed in the form of a graph rather than a table. Since a graph is based completely on the tabled scores, it does not contain any new information. However, a graph presents the data pictorially, which often makes it easier to see the important features of the data such as the *general shape*, the *spread* and the location of the *centre* of the distribution.

Frequency distributions of *nominal* or *ordinal* data are usually plotted using pie graphs or bar graphs. With this sort of data the intervals, or categories, are considered to be quite distinct and separate. For example, the type of blood you have, the football team you support, the car you drive, your favourite television program; all these variables are characterised by distinct categories rather than intervals. You have either Type A blood or some other type of blood. You support Collingwood, or you do not support Collingwood. The use of bar graphs or pie graphs emphasises the fact the data is being considered in discrete categories, rather than using a continuous scale such as heights, weights, test scores, etc.

When constructing a pie graph the angle of each sector will vary according to the *relative frequency* of each category. For example, if 10% of the data falls into a particular category then 10% of the pie graph should be marked accordingly. If we think of the pie graph as a circle with 360°, the respective segment of the pie graph should measure 36° (10% of 360°). Relative frequencies are found by dividing the actual frequency by the total of the frequencies. In effect, this will give the *proportion* of the data associated with each particular category.

EXAMPLE **2.3**

Construct a suitable pie graph for the following data on blood types.

Raw Data   O O A B A O A A A O A A A B A A O O A AB
B O B O O A O O A A O A A A O A O O AB

Solution
First, arrange the data into a suitable frequency table and calculate the appropriate relative frequencies:

Blood type	Frequency	Relative frequency
A	18	$18/40 = 45\%$
O	16	$16/40 = 40\%$
B	4	$4/40 = 10\%$
AB	2	$2/40 = 5\%$
Total	40	

EXAMPLE **2.3**   **cont.**

Second, calculate the respective angles for the pie graph:

45% of 360° is 162° for type A; 40% of 360° is 144° for type O;
10% of 360° is 36° for type B; 5% of 360° is 18° for type AB

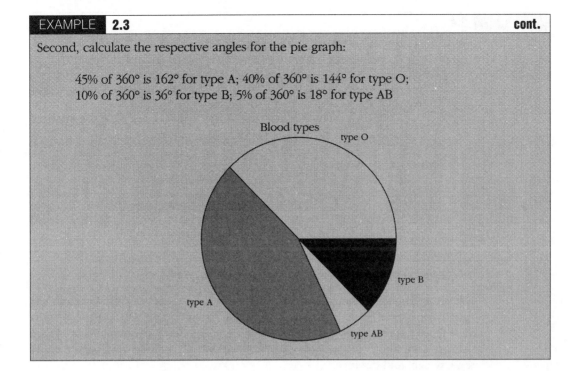

Bar graphs, on the other hand, are slightly easier to construct. Each category is represented by a single bar, the length of which is determined by the frequencies within each of the categories. The bars representing each category in a bar graph do not touch each other, which emphasises the fact that the data is being considered in discrete categories. The bars may be arranged either horizontally or vertically, and while order is not necessarily important, the categories are usually arranged in order of magnitude. This makes for easier reading and interpretation of the data. In the next example, based upon the blood types of 40 patients, the bars are placed horizontally and arranged in ascending order from the top of the graph to the bottom of the graph.

EXAMPLE **2.4**

Construct a bar graph based upon the blood-type data in Example 2.1.

Raw Data   O O A B A O A A A O A A A B A A O O A AB
              B O B O O A O O A A O O A A A O A O O AB

Solution

Blood type	Frequency
A	18
O	16
B	4
AB	2
Total	40

EXAMPLE   2.4   cont.

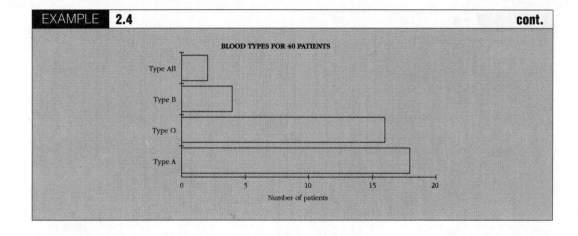

BLOOD TYPES FOR 40 PATIENTS

2.3   *Histograms and frequency polygons*

Data that has been obtained using interval or ratio scales of measurement are usually presented in the form of a histogram, or line graph. Data of this form is sometimes referred to as *continuous data*, because often measurements are made using a continuous scale. Examples of these would include variables such as time, weight and distance.

In Example 2.5, the distinct categories that were a feature of the previous blood-type examples above are replaced by class intervals (ie ranges of values). These intervals are plotted on the horizontal axis, beginning and terminating at the lower and upper limits of each interval. Note that the *areas* of the bars represent the frequencies or relative frequencies of the data with respect to each of the intervals: the heights of the histogram bars represent frequencies only when the intervals are of equal width. Since the intervals are continuous, the vertical bars touch each other.

EXAMPLE   2.5

(a)

The age distribution of respondents to a psychologist's survey is given below; present this data as a histogram.

Age	Respondents
15 – 19	515
20 – 29	177
30 – 49	204
50 – 79	100
Total	996

EXAMPLE 2.5   cont.

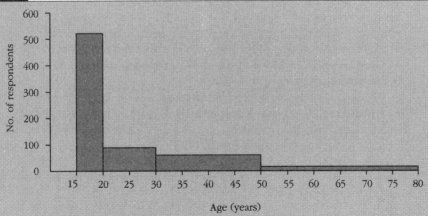

(b)

The following times in seconds represent the time required for a particular drug to take effect. Arrange these times into a suitable graphic display.

Raw Data   78 37 99 66 90 79 80 89 68 57 71 78 53 81 77 58 93
            79 88 76 60 77 49 92 83 80 74 69 90 62 84 64 73 48
            75 98 42 75 84 87 65 59 63 86 95 55 70 62 85 72

Solution

First, arrange the times into a suitable table.

Times (sec)	Frequency
30 – 39	1
40 – 49	3
50 – 59	5
60 – 69	9
70 – 79	14
80 – 89	11
90 – 99	7
Total	50

Now construct the appropriate histogram.

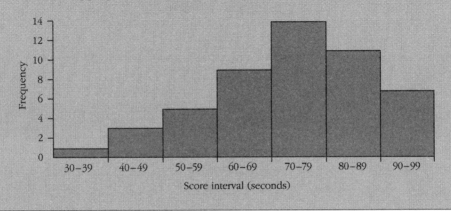

In this example the interval sizes are all the same (10) and there is no overlap between any of the intervals. Any particular value can be placed into *one* interval only. A time of 49.4 seconds, for example, would be placed into the interval 40 – 49. However, a time of 49.6 seconds would be placed into the interval 50 – 59. This is because 49.4 rounds down to 49, while 49.6 rounds up to 50. (A score of 49.5 can be either rounded down to 49 or rounded up to 50. With scores like this, be consistent one way or the other.)

Frequency polygons are an alternative way of presenting information contained in a histogram. They are constructed by plotting the *midpoints* of each of the intervals against their respective frequencies, or relative frequencies, and then connecting the midpoints with straight lines. The straight lines have no significance, but are merely an aid for the eye. The frequency polygon is made to touch the horizontal axis at both ends of the distribution by adding intervals with zero frequencies at each end.

EXAMPLE 2.6

Construct a suitable frequency polygon for the drug reaction times data below.

Raw Scores   78 37 99 66 90 79 80 89 68 57 71 78 53 81 77 58 93
              79 88 76 60 77 49 92 83 80 74 69 90 62 84 64 73 48
              75 98 42 75 84 87 65 59 63 86 95 55 70 62 85 72

Solution
First, arrange the values into a table with suitable midpoint values.

Score interval	Frequency	Midpoint
30 – 39	1	34.5
40 – 49	3	44.5
50 – 59	5	54.5
60 – 69	9	64.5
70 – 79	14	74.5
80 – 89	11	84.5
90 – 99	7	94.5
Total	50	

Now construct the appropriate frequency polygon.

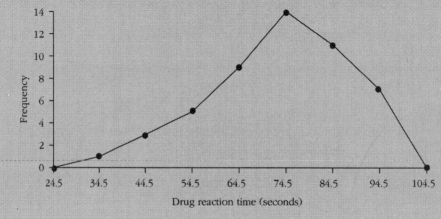

Drug reaction time (seconds)

Note that the histogram displays the values as though they were evenly spread through the interval, whereas the frequency polygon displays the values as if they were concentrated at the midpoint of each interval. Any interpretation of the line segments between each of the midpoints can therefore be only approximate.

Frequency polygons and histograms impart the same information; the choice between them is largely a matter of personal preference. The histogram is probably a little easier to interpret, but the stepwise bars tend to obscure the shape of the distribution. The frequency polygon is preferred when two or more sets of data are represented in the same graph, since superimposed histograms, even markedly different ones, are difficult to interpret.

2.4 Line graphs

Unlike the frequency polygon, a line graph does allow for accurate interpretation of the line segments between any two adjacent points. As the following example shows, these graphs are constructed on the basis of *paired data points* rather than frequencies. A line graph depicts the relationship between *two* variables, whereas a frequency polygon is concerned with frequencies that relate to only *one* variable.

EXAMPLE 2.7

A cup of coffee was made with boiling water and left to cool for 10 minutes. The temperature of the cup of coffee was recorded at one minute intervals. The resulting data is given below. Plot a suitable line graph for this data and determine what the temperature was 6.5 minutes after initially pouring the boiling water into the cup.

Raw Data	Time since pouring (mins)	1	2	3	4	5	6	7	8	9	10
	Temperature (°C)	98	90	84	78	74	70	67	64	62	60

Solution
Each pair of data points is plotted on a set of X–Y axes. In this case temperature is the dependent variable, and is therefore placed on the vertical axis.

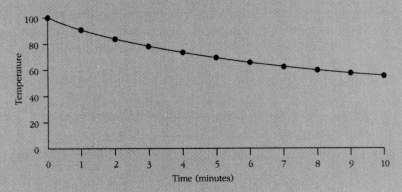

From the line graph it can be seen that at the 6.5 minute mark the temperature of the cup of coffee would probably have been about 68 or 69°C.

An exception to the above is the cumulative frequency polygon (or *ogive*), a line graph used to represent single variable data. This type of graph is used to show the number, proportion, or percentage of scores, that lie at or below the upper limit of each class interval. Instead of plotting frequencies against midpoints of class intervals, we plot cumulative frequencies against the upper limits of each interval. The vertical axis usually represents cumulative frequency (proportion, or percentage), while the upper limits of the score intervals are plotted on the horizontal axis. A cumulative percentage frequency polygon for the drug reaction times is shown in Example 2.8. As is often the case the cumulative frequency line graph has a characteristic S shape. The S shape occurs whenever there are more scores in the middle of the frequency polygon than at the extremes.

EXAMPLE 2.8

Construct a cumulative frequency polygon for the following drug reaction time data.

Raw Data	78	37	99	66	90	79	80	89	68	57	71	78	53	81	77	58	93
	79	88	76	60	77	49	92	83	80	74	69	90	62	84	64	73	48
	75	98	42	75	84	87	65	59	63	86	95	55	70	62	85	72	

Solution
First, arrange the data values into a table with an additional column containing cumulative frequencies.

Score interval	Frequency	Cumulative count
30 – 39	1	1 = 2%
40 – 49	3	4 = 8%
50 – 59	5	9 = 18%
60 – 69	9	18 = 36%
70 – 79	14	32 = 64%
80 – 89	11	43 = 86%
90 – 99	7	50 = 100%
Total	50	

Second, construct the cumulative frequency polygon by plotting the cumulative percentages against the upper limits of each interval.

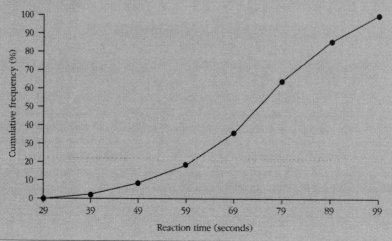

Practical statistics for the health sciences

2.5 Percentile points and percentile ranks

From graphs such as the ogive in Example 2.8 we can easily determine the proportion of the data that lie above or below particular data values. The proportion of scores less than or equal to 55, for example, represents the *percentile rank* of the score 55. In this case it would be approximately 15%. In other words, the percentile rank of a score of 55 is 15, because 15% of the scores are less than or equal to 55.

On the other hand, if we are interested in a certain proportion of scores being less than or equal to a particular data value, then that particular value is referred to as a *percentile point*. For example, the 25th percentile point is a point such that 25% of the data values are less than or equal to this particular point. In this case the 25th percentile point would be represented by a score of about 63 or 64. (Plotting the data on graph paper would enable a more accurate interpretation.)

2.6 Stem-and-leaf displays

In recent years a technique known as the *stem-and-leaf display* has become very popular, and it is well suited for computer application. This technique, very simple to create and use, is a combination of a graphic technique and a sorting technique. (Sorting data means making a list of the data in rank order according to numerical value.) The data values themselves are used to do this sorting. Stems consist of the leading digits of the data, while the leaves consist of the trailing digits. For example, the numerical data value 458 might be split into a stem of 45 tens and a leaf of 8 units. This would normally be displayed as follows:

Stem	Leaf (unit = 1)
45	8

Alternatively, the stem may well consist of the hundreds digit, ie 4, and the leaf comprising the tens digit, but rounded to the nearest ten, ie 6. This would give:

Stem	Leaf (unit = 10)
4	6

In this instance the actual data score of 458 is being represented by the rounded score of 460. Note that the leaf unit consists of *tens*, so the 6 represents 6 tens and not 6 units. The choice of the leaf unit depends upon the context of the data.

Stem-and-leaf displays group the data so that patterns are easily seen but with very little loss of the detail inherent in the original data. It is important that the digits are set out neatly so that the shape of the distribution becomes apparent. In the example below the first digit of each score has been used as the stem, while the second digit has been used as the leaf. In other words, a leaf unit = 1 has been chosen. The leaves have also been *ordered*. This is the preferred form for these displays. Notice how the setting out of the leaves highlights the shape of the data.

EXAMPLE **2.9**

Construct a stem-and-leaf display to represent the following data, which comprises the number of heartbeats per minute for a group of 20 students.

Raw Data	82	74	88	66	58	74	78	84	96	76
	62	68	72	92	86	76	52	76	82	78

Solution

Stem	Leaf (unit = 1)
5	2 8
6	2 6 8
7	2 4 4 6 6 6 8 8
8	2 2 4 6 8
9	2 6

The basic steps involved in constructing a stem-and-leaf display are:

1   Arrange the scores in numerical order.

2   Separate each observation into a suitable stem and leaf.

3   List the stems vertically in increasing order from top to bottom.

4   Draw a vertical line to the right of the stems then place the leaves to the right of the line.

An important advantage of a stem-and-leaf display over a histogram is that the display provides all of the information that is contained in a histogram while preserving the value of the individual scores.

2.7   *The pros and cons of grouping data*

Grouping scores into class intervals of size greater than 1 has several disadvantages. Firstly, some information is inevitably lost. For example, we may know that four scores occur in the interval 54 – 56, but we do not know their individual values. They may all be 55s, or they may be spread equally from 54 to 56. If we do not have access to the original data then we are not in a position to know what the original scores were.

A second disadvantage is that the rules used to construct grouped frequency distributions do not always produce unique distributions. For any set of data, only one ungrouped frequency distribution can be constructed, but for grouped frequency distributions, there is often a choice between two or more class interval sizes. In such cases, the shape of the frequency distribution can depend on the size of the class interval chosen. This problem was demonstrated in Section 2.1 when discussing frequency tables.

The disadvantages of the loss of information and lack of uniqueness resulting from grouping scores into class intervals of size greater than 1 must be weighed against the simplicity achieved by grouping. If the spread of scores is large, a grouped frequency distribution is much more easily interpreted. Also, the construction of a grouped frequency distribution is necessary if a graph for a quantitative variable is to be made, since the first step in making such a graph often involves grouping the data points into suitable intervals. Grouping was used to minimise the labour required in computing statistics, but the advent of hand-held calculators and computers eliminated this use for grouped frequency distributions.

2.8   *Minitab*

In this book we will assume that access to the statistical package Minitab is readily available. Minitab comprises a worksheet for data storage and a vocabulary of more than 200 commands and subcommands. Information on any command, or subcommand, can be obtained from the system itself by typing HELP followed by the command or subcommand in question. All commands are typed *after* the Minitab prompt MTB >.

To demonstrate the usefulness of computer packages such as Minitab, a short analysis of some data will be done using some of Minitab's basic commands. The Minitab commands used have been put into bold type as have any other entries made by the user (data input, punctuation, subcommands, etc.). Responses to these commands and entries have been left in normal type. Note that Minitab automatically chooses the most appropriate interval and/or scale for the displays requested. These can be changed if required.

EXAMPLE	2.10

The following final examination marks (maximum = 60) were obtained by students studying statistics at university level.

Student Marks	10	13	22	26	16	23	35	53	17	32	41	35	24	23	27	16	20	60
	48	43	52	31	17	20	33	18	23	8	24	15	26	46	30	19	22	13
	22	14	21	39	28	43	37	15	11	20	25	9	15	21	21	25	34	10
	23	29	28	18	17	24	16	26	7	12	28	20	36	16	14	18	16	57

Produce histogram, dotplot and stem-and-leaf displays for the above data.

```
MTB > set c1
DATA> 10 13 22 26 16 23 35 53 17 32 41 35 24 23 27 16 20 60 48 43
DATA> 52 31 17 20 33 18 23 8 24 15 26 46 30 19 22 13 22 14 21 39
DATA> 28 43 37 15 20 11 25 9 15 21 21 25 34 10 23 29 28 18 17 24
DATA> 16 26 7 12 28 20 36 16 14 18 16 57
DATA> end
MTB > name c1 'Exam'
MTB > hist c1
```

EXAMPLE 2.10   cont.

```
Histogram of Exam   N = 72
 Midpoint   Count
     5      1  *
    10      6  ******
    15     15  ***************
    20     14  **************
    25     13  *************
    30      7  *******
    35      6  ******
    40      2  **
    45      3  ***
    50      2  **
    55      2  **
    60      1  *
```

MTB > **dotplot c1**

```
                    .
              .:.. :..:. . .
         ...:.::::::::.::::::::.:........:. . . :  .. . ..  . .
      -----+---------+---------+---------+---------+---------+-Exam
           10        20        30        40        50        60
```

MTB > **stem c1**

```
Stem-and-leaf of Exam    N = 72
Leaf Unit = 1.0

   3   0 789
  11   1 00123344
  26   1 555666667778889
 (17)  2 00001112223333444
  29   2 5566678889
  19   3 01234
  14   3 55679
   9   4 133
   6   4 68
   4   5 23
   2   5 7
   1   6 0
```

1 The graph below illustrates the number of cases of Ross River virus reported in Victoria in 1992/93 based on 8 regions.

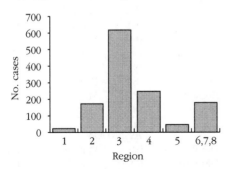

(a) Why has a bar graph been used for this data?

(b) Which region had the highest incidence of this disease?

The graph below shows the number of reported cases in 1990/91.

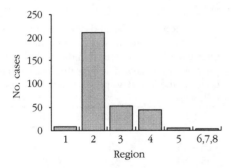

(c) Which region(s) had the lowest incidence of the virus?

(d) Which region experienced the greatest change between 1990/91 and 1992/93?

(e) Express this change as a percentage change.

2 Peak flow meters are commonly used to assess the state of asthma sufferers.

(a) Estimate the mean peak flow rate for those children who are 150 cm tall.

MEAN PEAK FLOW RATES FOR CHILDREN

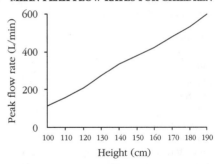

(b) Children whose peak flow rate is 75 L/min less than the mean rate for their height may be considered to be 'ill'. For children 110–120 cm tall, what would these lower limits be?

(c) A child in my class is 170 cm tall and is blowing a peak flow rate of 420 L/min. Does she need medical help?

3 One hundred athletes took part in a prolonged repetitive exercise program. The following is the distribution of the number of times that athletes needed to stop for longer than 10 seconds.

Number of stops	Number of athletes
0	23
1	25
2	19
3	14
4	11
5	5
6	2
7	1

(a) What percentage of the group had to stop more than 5 times?

(b) What is the relative frequency of the athletes that stopped twice or less?

(c) Draw a histogram to represent this data.

4 In Victoria in 1989–90 the following data was estimated for the use of sunscreens.

Usually use sunscreen	Number of people (thousands)
SPF 2–3	3.7
SPF 4–7	115.7
SPF 8–14	247.3
SPF ≥15	1923.0
Depends/varies	55.3
Don't know	271.8
Protected by clothes, hat etc.	102.6
Not exposed to strong sun	287.9
Not protected	1356.1

Convert this information to percentages and display it using a graph.

5 On 30 September 1991 there were 8559 persons registered at the CES as unemployed. Of this number, 1379 had been unemployed for less than three months, 1800 had been unemployed for more than three months, but less than six months, 1513 had been unemployed for more than six but less than nine months, 1220 had been unemployed for between nine and twelve months, and 2647 had been unemployed for more than twelve months. Present this data using a table and then an appropriate graphical display.

6 Height has long been regarded as an important asset for a league footballer. Use the information below (in cm) to construct back-to-back stem-and-leaf plots then comment on whether you think that height may have contributed to Collingwood's defeat of Essendon in the 1990 AFL grand final. Place stems in centre, with leaves for Collingwood to the left of the stem and leaves for Essendon to the right.

COLLINGWOOD			
Christian	193	Millane	192
Gayfer	183	Wright	178
Kerrison	178	Shaw	170
Morwood	191	Manson	194
Kelly	189	Banks	185
Crosisca	189	Barwick	173
Starcevich	193	Turner	183
Daicos	184	Brown	183
Russell	180	Monkhorst	203
McGuane	185	Francis	170

ESSENDON			
Daniher	191	Van Der Haar	192
Hamilton	189	Cransberg	190
Thompson	175	Harvey	179
Daniher	188	Daniher	193
Grenvold	183	Salmon	206
O'Donnell	181	Sporn	186
Somerville	198	Ezard	172
Anderson	188	Madden	198
Kickett	183	Watson	185
Long	178	Bewick	178

7 One hundred females and one hundred males from each age group were questioned about their use of non-prescription drugs during the previous four days. The reported use of analgesics in the four days prior to interview was as follows:

Age	Females	Males
15 – 24	25	19
25 – 44	30	21
45 – 54	32	21
55 – 64	30	25
65+	32	25

Present this data graphically in a way which will allow comparison between males and females and between age groups.

8 The following table shows the ages of 50 clients attending aerobics classes at a fitness centre.

Age	Number of clients
20 - 29	11
30 - 39	18
40 - 49	9
50 - 59	8
60 - 69	4

Graph this data and describe the distribution.

9 A case report on child cyclist accidents in a certain area yielded the following data:

Age	Number of accidents
5	2
6	10
7	5
8	4
9	5
10	8
11	8
12	14
13	12
14	12
15	16
16	11

(a) Extend the frequency table to show relative and cumulative frequencies.
(b) Construct an ogive for the above data.
(c) Fifty per cent of the children who had accidents were under .... years of age.
(d) Children less than 10 years of age contributed .... per cent of the accidents.
(e) Twenty five per cent of children who had accidents were aged .... and over.

CHAPTER OUTLINE

CHAPTER THREE

Describing Distributions

LEARNING OBJECTIVES

After studying this chapter you should be able to:

- use appropriate vocabulary to describe the shape of a distribution;
- correctly calculate the mean, median and mode of a small set of data;
- choose an appropriate measure of central tendency for any given set of data;
- locate other key points in a distribution, ie percentiles and quartiles;
- construct and interpret a box-and-whisker plot;
- correctly calculate the range, interquartile range, variance and standard deviation for a set of data;
- use Minitab to obtain descriptive statistics and examine the shape of a set of data;
- identify and deal with outliers; and
- write a detailed statistical description of a set of data, including shape and appropriate measures of location and variability.

Having gathered some raw data we are usually interested in *describing* it in some way. Describing the data is a part of what is called *exploratory data analysis*. This is a worthwhile step prior to embarking upon more sophisticated analyses of the data. By having a good look at the data first of all, you may find that further analysis is not warranted, or that a different pattern or relationship from the one expected may be apparent.

Generally, exploratory procedures are best handled by computer packages like Minitab, where it is both quick and easy to obtain simple graphs of the data as well as some basic statistics such as averages, standard deviations and maximum and minimum values. The identification of any *unusual* values is also important at this stage. These unusual values are called *outliers*, and may simply represent extreme values in the data set. They may, however, also represent errors, either when the data was collected or when it was put into the computer or calculator.

3.1 Shape

The shape of a distribution is determined by looking at a graph (frequency polygon, histogram, or stem-and-leaf) of the distribution. Some of the more common terms that we use to describe distributions are shown in Figure 3.1. The shape of a distribution is important because it will determine the *mathematical model* that we can use to further investigate the distribution. If we know which model is appropriate then we are in a position to use any of the mathematical properties that are associated with that model.

Of particular importance is the bell-shaped or mound-shaped distribution shown in Figure 3.1. This shape is often referred to as the *normal distribution*. There are many instances where this distribution seems to occur naturally. For example, many measurements made with respect to people appear to have this sort of distribution (height, weight, intelligence, and so on). Also, the dimensions of components made in manufacturing processes can have normal distributions.

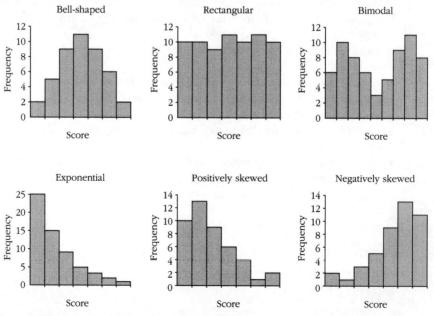

Figure 3.1 Common descriptions of frequency distributions.

Some other examples might include the following:

- The number of times that each of the numbers 1 to 45 have occurred in the weekly Tattslotto draws over a long time will be *rectangular* (or *uniform*).
- Height, and times for running or swimming for adults will show *bimodal* distributions — one peak for males and one for females.
- Waiting times between phone calls, or between arrivals of accident cases, are likely to show *exponential* distributions.
- People's salaries, house prices, student performance on a difficult test, and the number of cars passing by a certain point on the road in a given amount of time, are likely to be *positively skewed*.
- Student performance on an easy test is likely to be *negatively skewed*.

3.2   *Measures of central tendency*

In order to summarise the key features of a set of data we must be able to quote some typical (or average) value which will indicate the location of the centre of the distribution. For example, when planning a holiday to a distant place it is common to check the average maximum and minimum temperatures experienced at that time of the year. If you find that the average daily maximum temperature is 25°C then you know to pack T-shirts and shorts. There is no expectation that the temperature will reach 25°C every day; rather that it will be something close to that. The average temperature statistic indicates the sort of temperature that you might expect.

There are several kinds of measures ordinarily known as *averages*, and each one gives a different picture of the data it is called on to represent. Consider, for example, the maximum temperatures (in °C) reached on each of 10 consecutive days in September on the Gold Coast in Queensland:

24.0   29.0   27.5   26.75   25.25   21.5   21.5   21.5   21.5   25.5

If you were intending to holiday at the Gold Coast next September, a question you may well ask is: What is the average temperature likely to be? In other words, how warm can you expect the days to be at that time of the year? There are three commonly used statistics that are used to measure, or indicate, the centre of a distribution: the mean, the median and the mode.

We will consider each one of these central measures as they would apply to this example.

The mean

The arithmetic mean is the most common form of average. It is obtained simply by the following process:

1   Add all of the scores together.

2   Divide by the total number of scores.

In the example above, the average of the 10 daily temperatures is 24.4°C.

When we calculate such measures for sample data, the measures are called *sample statistics*, but when calculations are based upon an entire population they are known as *population parameters*. Symbolically, we distinguish between sample statistics and population parameters by using Roman letters for statistics and Greek letters for parameters. Therefore we define the mean as follows:

$$\text{sample mean} \qquad \bar{x} = \frac{\Sigma x}{n}$$

$$\text{population mean} \quad \mu = \frac{\Sigma x}{N}$$

The Greek letter Σ (sigma) is used to represent *the sum of*, x is used to represent each data value (ie maximum daily temperature), n represents the size of the sample and N is the size of the population.

The mean represents the centre of a distribution in the sense that the sum of the amounts by which the higher temperatures *exceed* the mean is exactly the same as the sum of the amounts by which the lower temperatures are less than the mean. Put in another way, the sum of the differences between the mean and each temperature is equal to zero. This will always be the case. Algebraically we write this as follows:

$$\Sigma(x - \bar{x}) = 0$$

The median

The median is the point which divides the data set in half. The median locates the middle of the distribution in the sense that a particular observation is *equally likely* to be above or below the median. (That is, half the values are above the median and half are below.) To determine the median of a set of data, the following steps apply:

1   Arrange the data into either ascending, or descending, order.

2   Locate the point below which half the values lie.

For 10 data values, as in the Gold Coast temperature data we looked at earlier, there is no exact middle value as such. To obtain the median in this case we average the two central values (ie the fifth and sixth temperatures). The median therefore works out to be 24.625°C, which in this case is more than the mean.

29.0	27.5	26.75	25.5	25.25	24.0	21.5	21.5	21.5	21.5

$$\qquad\qquad\qquad\qquad \downarrow \qquad\quad \downarrow$$
$$\qquad\qquad\qquad\qquad \text{5th} \qquad \text{6th}$$
$$\qquad\qquad\qquad\qquad \text{score} \quad\; \text{score}$$

$$\frac{25.25 + 24}{2} = \frac{49.25}{2} = 24.625$$

Figure 3.2 Calculation of the median for temperature data.

The median does not depend upon extreme values, and is most useful if the tails of the distribution are incompletely specified by open-ended intervals such as 40.0+°C.

The mode

The data value that occurs most frequently is called the mode. In the temperature example, 21.5°C was the temperature that occurred most often, so it is the mode for that data set. If no two or more days recorded the same temperature, then

Practical statistics for the health sciences

there would have been no mode for this sample. On the other hand, it is possible for a distribution to have more than one mode, as in *bimodal* or *multimodal* distributions. The mode is easy to calculate, and it is the only one of the three measures appropriate for categorical data because it describes the most typical case.

Choosing an appropriate central measure

So we have three different 'averages', each valid, correct, and informative in its own way. But they do differ, and depending upon the context within which they are being used they can present differing views of the centre of the distribution:

mean	24.4°C
median	24.625°C
mode	21.5°C

Which temperature would you choose to report if you were employed as a tourist officer by the Gold Coast city council? By reporting the *median* you would be giving the most favourable picture for daily maximum temperatures in the area. However, by reporting the *mean* or the *mode* you are presenting a less favourable image. The final choice can often be influenced by the context of the situation. For example, people from the colder southern climates would most likely be happy with any temperature above 20°C, whereas those from hot northern climates may be more attracted by the modal temperature.

Even though both the mean and mode are correct as measures of central tendency, they can be misleading if a distribution is markedly skewed. The most appropriate measure for such a distribution is the median. This example illustrates just one of the ways in which statistics can be used to mislead the unwary.

When dealing with averages there are several things worth remembering. First, when people use the term average they might just mean *typical* and not be referring to a statistic at all. If a statistic has been used it will most commonly have been the arithmetic mean, but not always. Therefore you should check carefully to find out what information you have actually been given, ie mean, median or mode.

Second, consider the data referred to and see whether or not the average used is appropriate, or in fact if it is meaningful. For example, when numbers are used as *labels*, calculating a mean is not appropriate because it will have no sensible meaning.

The mean is the most common measure of central tendency. One desirable characteristic of the mean that should be mentioned here is its *stability*. If several samples are taken from one large set of data, and the mode, median and mean are calculated for each sample, the mean tends to *vary less* from sample to sample than the median or the mode. Nonetheless, it is true that a single outlier (an unusually high or low data value) can unduly affect the value of the mean while leaving the mode and the median unchanged.

In physical terms the mean represents the centre of gravity (that is, the balancing point) of a distribution. Imagine a group of people standing on a flat platform which in turn is balanced at a single point. The mean can be thought of as the balancing point. If any person decides to move the balancing point changes. This is similar to a raft floating on water. We all know what happens when somebody starts jumping up and down or tries to get back onto the raft. The mean is that value which *balances* the distribution, which in the Gold Coast temperature case would be the value 24.4°C.

Comparing means, medians and modes

In any distribution, if the mean and the median coincide (ie mean = median) then the distribution will be *symmetrical.* If the distribution is skewed then the mean will tend to be pulled towards the direction of the skew. This relationship between the three measures of central tendency, with respect to the shape of the distribution, can be seen in Figure 3.3.

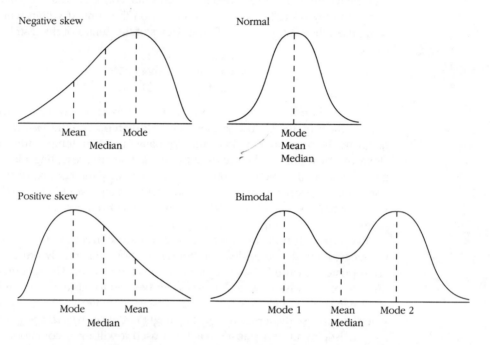

Figure 3.3 The shape of a distribution affects the positions of mean, median and mode.

The choice of whether to report the mean, median, or the mode will depend upon the message to be conveyed to the reader or the consumer. Distorted interpretations of data can be misleading to consumers, particularly when dealing with skewed distributions. Consider the following situation, in which the distribution is positively skewed:

The salaries of staff at a particular workplace had the following characteristics:

mean = $500   median = $450   mode = $400

In negotiating a new contract for these workers, the local union representative might report the modal wage in order to support a request for a wage increase. However, if you were on the other side of the negotiating table, you might cite the mean, a higher figure, in arguing against the need for an increase.

Both the mean and the mode can be misleading when the distribution is markedly skewed; a more appropriate measure for skewed distributions is the median.

Practical statistics for the health sciences

EXAMPLE 3.1

The following data was gathered from a sample of 20 adults who considered themselves to be regular smokers. Each person was asked to smoke a cigarette while sitting watching television. Upon finishing the cigarette their pulse rate (per minute) was recorded. Find the mean pulse rate for the group, as well as the median and mode.

Raw Data	72	84	75	73	69	76	70	82	77	84
	90	73	72	75	78	81	66	75	78	73

Solution
Sort the data into ascending or descending order. This will make it easy to determine the median and the mode.

66 69 70 72 72 73 73 73 75 75 75 76 77 78 78 81 82 84 84 90

(a) Finding the mean: $\bar{x} = \dfrac{\sum x}{n}$, $\sum x = 1523$, so $\bar{x} = \dfrac{1523}{20} = 76.15$

(b) Finding the median: The median lies half way between the 10th and 11th values in this case, ie between 75 and 75. Therefore the median is 75.

(c) Finding the mode: The values 73 and 75 occur most often, so they are the modes.

Trimmed means

Sometimes a set of data would be approximately symmetrical if it were not for one or two unusually high or low values. In this case the best solution might be to trim these extreme values and calculate the mean of the remaining data. This is then called a trimmed mean. This approach is often used when judging events such as gymnastics or diving, where the highest and lowest scores are ignored and a competitor's final score is based upon the trimmed data. This method supposedly overcomes the bias that judges may have for particular competitors.

If a 5% trimmed mean is calculated, then the lower 5% *and* the upper 5% of the data values are ignored, and the average of the remaining 90% of the data set is calculated. So a 5% trimmed mean is in fact the mean of the middle 90% of the data values. In the same way, a 10% trimmed mean is the mean of the middle 80% of the data.

EXAMPLE 3.2

Calculate a 5% trimmed mean for the pulse-rate data based upon the sample of smokers used in Example 3.1.

Raw Data	72	84	75	73	69	76	70	82	77	84
	90	73	72	75	78	81	66	75	78	73

Solution
First remove the top and bottom 5% of the data. As 5% of 20 = 1, we remove the lowest value (66) and the highest value (90). This leaves the following:

EXAMPLE **3.2** **cont.**

69 70 72 72 73 73 73 75 75 75 76 77 78 78 81 82 84 84

Finding the trimmed mean: $\bar{x} = \dfrac{\Sigma x}{n}$, $\Sigma x = 1367$, so $\bar{x} = \dfrac{1367}{18} = 75.94$

3.3   *Percentiles and quartiles*

In Chapter 2, percentile points were defined as values on the score axis such that n% of the distribution is less than a particular point. Percentile points are sometimes used when describing distributions. For example, some of the more common percentile points used as standards for comparison of data sets are:

- the 0th percentile point (ie the minimum value);
- the 25th percentile point, also known as the *first quartile* or Q_1 (one-quarter of the distribution lies below this point);
- the 50th percentile point, also known as the median, and sometimes written P_{50} (half the distribution lies above this point and half lies below);
- the 75th percentile point, or the *third quartile*, Q_3 (three-quarters of the distribution lies below this point); and
- the 100th percentile point (ie the maximum value).

Of particular interest are the first and third quartiles, because half the data lies between these two points. Another way to think of these two points is to think of the middle 50% of the data lying between them. In Example 3.3, the middle 50% of the data lie between the points 72.5 and 79.5. Finding quartiles is quite straightforward for a sample of size 20, because you have 5 data values in each quarter. With more awkward sample sizes, like 17 or 29, use common sense, and be consistent when partitioning the data set into quarters.

EXAMPLE **3.3**

Find the first and third quartiles for the smokers' pulse-rate data below.

Raw Data   72   84   75   73   69   76   70   82   77   84
            90   73   72   75   78   81   66   75   78   73

Solution

First sort the data into ascending or descending order, then partition the data set into quarters.

66 69 70 72 72 73 73 73 75 75 75 76 77 78 78 81 82 84 84 90
            ↓   ↓   ↓

           Q_1 P_{50} Q_3

The first quartile is therefore halfway between the values 72 and 73, ie 72.5.
The third quartile lies halfway between the values 78 and 81, ie 79.5.

Box-and-whisker plots from Minitab

Box-and-whisker plots (or boxplots) use percentile points to provide a pictorial summary of both the centre *and* the spread of the data. As the name suggests, this method of describing data consists primarily of a drawing of a *box* with *whiskers* that extend from either end. The ends of the box are defined by the first and third quartiles, and the median is usually indicated by a mark inside the box. The whiskers extend from either end of the box by an amount no more than 1.5 times the spread of the box. The spread of the box is defined to be the difference between the first and the third quartiles, ie $Q_3 - Q_1$. Any data values that lie beyond the limit of the whiskers are considered to be outliers and are indicated as such. Minitab uses asterisks (*) or circles (o) to indicate outliers. The circle is used to indicate data values that lie more than three times the spread of the box from either end of the box. These are sometimes called *extreme outliers*.

In the following Minitab printout the pulse-rate data for the group of 20 smokers was entered into column 1 and named accordingly. The column was then printed, sorted, and printed again. Various descriptive statistics can be obtained with the one command, DESCRIBE. Notice that, as well as the mean, median, and trimmed mean, DESCRIBE also produces the minimum and maximum values, plus the first and third quartiles. From the boxplot that was requested note the values associated with the ends of the box, and with the median. In this instance there are no outliers indicated. The histogram produced by Minitab shows a positive skew to the data. The intervals were automatically selected by Minitab, which prints only the midpoints of the intervals. In this case Minitab chose an interval size of 4.

```
MTB > set c1
DATA> 72 84 75 73 69 76 70 82 77 84 90 73 72 75 78 81 66 75 78 73
DATA> end
MTB > name c1 'Pulse'
MTB > print c1


Pulse
  72   84   75   73   69   76   70   82   77   84   90   73   72
  75   78   81   66   75   78   73

MTB > sort c1 c2


MTB > print c2


C2
 66   69   70   72   72   73   73   73   75   75   75   76   77
 78   78   81   82   84   84   90

MTB > desc c1


             N      MEAN    MEDIAN     TRMEAN     STDEV   SEMEAN
Pulse       20     76.15     75.00      75.94      5.81     1.30


           MIN       MAX        Q1         Q3
Pulse     66.00     90.00     72.25      80.25
```

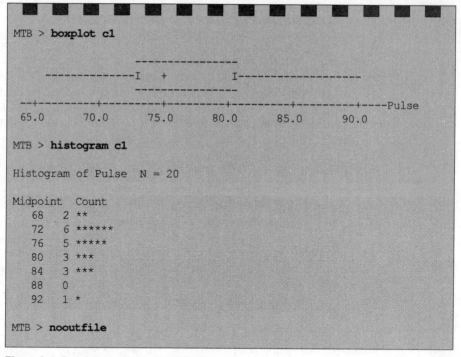

```
MTB > boxplot c1


                                -------------------
              ---------------I    +          I----------------------
                                -------------------

     --+----------+----------+----------+----------+----------+-----Pulse
     65.0       70.0       75.0       80.0       85.0       90.0

MTB > histogram c1

Histogram of Pulse   N = 20

Midpoint  Count
    68    2 **
    72    6 ******
    76    5 *****
    80    3 ***
    84    3 ***
    88    0
    92    1 *

MTB > nooutfile
```

Figure 3.4 Descriptive measures from Minitab.

3.5   *Measures of dispersion or spread*

An average, by itself, does not tell us everything that we might want to know about a particular data set. In the previous section box-and-whisker plots were introduced as pictorial representations of data indicating the positions of various points of interest, including the median. However, by indicating the positions of the various quartiles the box-and-whisker plot was able to give us some idea of the spread of the data in each quarter of the distribution. In addition to measures of central tendency it is often helpful to have some information about how the numbers vary.

Dispersion, or *variability*, has to do with how far the data values are spread apart. The statistics that we use most frequently to describe, or measure dispersion, include the range, interquartile range, variance and standard deviation.

The range

The range is the difference between the maximum and minimum scores in the distribution. While it is quick and easy to calculate, it provides only a crude measure of dispersion because it only measures the spread of the data in terms of the two extreme scores: it ignores the data values in the rest of the distribution. The range is useful, however, when *organisation* is important. This may be organising a data set into a table where values are grouped into intervals, or it may be organising what clothes you want to take with you to your holiday on the Gold Coast (ie the temperature range is important).

$$\text{range} = \text{maximum} - \text{minimum}$$

The range is used for quantitative variables, and is often reported with the mode. The great advantage of the range is its simplicity; it is easy to understand and to compute. As a result, it is used widely as a preliminary measure of dispersion. It also is used in deciding how to group data into a frequency distribution. For example, we can estimate the number and the size of class intervals in a trial-and-error fashion using the formula

$$\frac{\text{range}}{\text{desired interval size}} = \text{no. of intervals}$$

The major deficiency of the range is its poor sampling stability. The range ignores most of the data values. It is sensitive to just two values in the distribution, and consequently, it is not robust. The range also depends upon sample size. If samples are selected randomly from a population, the range will tend to be larger for larger samples because large samples are more likely to include extreme scores. These deficiencies tend to limit the range to descriptive applications.

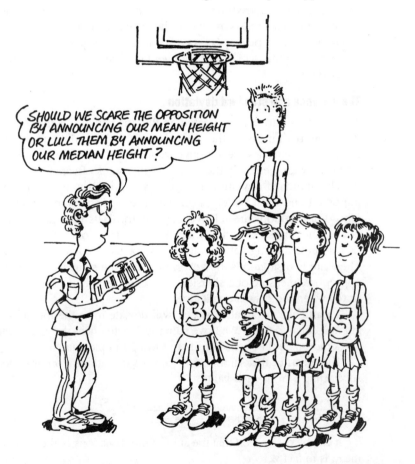

Source Adapted from Moore, D S 1985, *Statistics and Controversies*, W H Freeman & Co, New York, p 177

The interquartile range

The *interquartile range* (IQR) is the range of the middle two quartiles. That is, it is the difference between the first and third quartiles. Therefore the IQR represents the range of the middle 50% of the observations in a data set. We express this difference between the quartiles as follows:

$$IQR = Q_3 - Q_1$$

The IQR has been encountered previously because it was used to define the width of the 'box' in a box-and-whisker plot. It is a particularly useful measure of variation in data sets that are skewed, and also in data sets that have missing values or open-ended intervals. For these reasons the IQR is often reported along with the median, and as such shares the median's advantages and disadvantages. For example, the interquartile range is limited to descriptive applications with quantitative variables. Nevertheless, it is preferred over the standard deviation in two situations:

(a) Like the median, the IQR can be computed for open-ended distributions, particularly if the unknown scores lie above Q_3 or below Q_1. The IQR should be computed when the value of one or more extreme scores is unknown.

(b) The IQR is preferred over the standard deviation for skewed distributions. Recall that this measure is sensitive to the *number* but not to the *value* of scores lying above Q_3 and below Q_1. As a result the interquartile range is less influenced by the extreme scores in the longer tail of such a distribution than is the standard deviation.

The variance and standard deviation

These statistics are closely related, in that the variance is the square of the standard deviation. Both measure the *deviation* of the data values about the *mean*. Like the mean, these statistics are sensitive to all of the values in the data set, and because of this they are generally the preferred measures of variation.

The standard deviation is typically reported with the mean. It is the most important and most widely used measure of dispersion for quantitative variables whose distributions are relatively symmetrical. Its popularity is largely due to the fact that it varies less than other measures from one random sample to another (ie it shows sampling stability). It can also be used in many mathematical calculations. There are two situations, however, in which the standard deviation is not the most appropriate measure of dispersion. These are (a) when a distribution is very skewed or (b) when the data is qualitative.

A particular data value, say x, will deviate from the mean of its sample by an amount equal to $(x - \bar{x})$. If we sum these differences the result will always be zero. To demonstrate this, consider the following sample data: 6, 3, 8, 5, 3.

The mean of this sample is $\frac{25}{5} = 5$, so deviations from the mean are found by subtracting 5 from each value:

x	6	3	5	8	3
$x - 5$	$6 - 5 = 1$	$3 - 5 = -2$	$5 - 5 = 0$	$8 - 5 = 3$	$3 - 5 = -2$

It can be easily seen that the sum of the deviations of the scores from the sample mean is in fact zero:

$$1 + (-2) + 0 + 3 + (-2) = 0$$

If the deviation scores are first squared and then summed, this problem can be overcome because the negative differences become positive when squared. In other words, we are considering the *magnitude* of the squared differences. This results in the following:

Practical statistics for the health sciences

$$(1)^2 + (-2)^2 + (0)^2 + (3)^2 + (-2)^2 = 1 + 4 + 0 + 9 + 4 = 18$$

Algebraically we write this as $\Sigma(x - \bar{x})^2 = 18$, and we refer to it as the *sum of the squared deviations about the mean*, or simply the *sum of squares*. We divide by one less than the sample size to get the sample variance, which is denoted by s^2. So in this simple example the variance is:

$$s^2 = \tfrac{18}{4} = 4.5$$

By taking the square root of this value we have the sample standard deviation:

$$s = \sqrt{4.5} = 2.12$$

These sample statistics can be written algebraically as follows:

sample variance $\qquad\qquad s^2 = \dfrac{\Sigma(x - \bar{x})^2}{n - 1}$

sample standard deviation $\quad s = \sqrt{\dfrac{\Sigma(x - \bar{x})^2}{n - 1}}$

At this point we must distinguish between a sample and a population, because slightly different formulae apply. For populations we divide by N, which is the total size of the population, but for samples we divide by $n - 1$, which is one less than the sample size. The population parameters are then defined as

population variance $\qquad\qquad \sigma^2 = \dfrac{\Sigma(x - \mu)^2}{N}$

population standard deviation $\quad \sigma = \sqrt{\dfrac{\Sigma(x - \mu)^2}{N}}$

The Greek letter μ designates the population mean in the formulae above. Dividing the sum of squares by N is equivalent to finding the *average squared deviation* of the values about the population mean. When dealing with samples, dividing by n results in a *biased* estimate of the true population variance. To remove this bias, sample variances are calculated using $n-1$ as the denominator.

The standard deviation measures variation from the mean of the sample or population exactly as the formulae above set out. These formulae can present calculation problems, particularly when the value of the mean is an approximation or has been rounded. Each time the rounded mean is used in a calculation the answer will also be an approximation, ie there is a rounding error. Each difference between a data value and the mean is squared, further adding to the rounding error, and after many calculations this error accumulates. Algebraic techniques can be used to produce alternative versions of the formulae which circumvent this problem.

By expanding the brackets and simplifying the result, the following can be shown to be true:

$$\Sigma(x - \bar{x})^2 = \Sigma x^2 - \dfrac{(\Sigma x)^2}{n}$$

So s then becomes

$$s = \sqrt{\dfrac{\sum x^2 - \dfrac{(\sum x)^2}{n}}{n-1}}$$

or better still,

$$s = \sqrt{\dfrac{n\sum x^2 - (\sum x)^2}{n(n-1)}}$$

Using the formulae on page 43 makes use of the raw scores, thereby minimising any error associated with rounding the mean.

Checking calculations

When calculating standard deviations there are three ways to check on the sometimes quite tedious calculations.

1   A rough guide is that the ratio of the *range* to the standard deviation is rarely smaller than 2 or greater than 6.

2   By definition, it is impossible to obtain a *negative* value for the sum of squares.

3   Be aware of the difference between the two quantities $\sum x^2$ and $(\sum x)^2$. The first term represents the sum of the scores *after* each has been squared. The second term represents the square of the sum of all of the scores.

EXAMPLE **3.4**

A student kept a record of the number of additional hours per week spent studying statistics for one semester. The following weekly scores were recorded.

Raw Data   11.6 10 11.4 12.6 7.6 7.8 5 5 10.2 5 10.6 14.2 14.6 15.4

Determine the following statistics for the above data:
(a) mean (b) median (c) IQR (d) range (e) variance (f) standard deviation.

Solution   Ranking the above scores, we get the following:

5.0 5.0 5.0 7.6 7.8 10 10.2 10.6 11.4 11.6 12.6 14.2 14.6 15.4
$\qquad\qquad\quad\downarrow\qquad\qquad\qquad\downarrow\qquad\qquad\qquad\qquad\quad\downarrow$
$\qquad\qquad\quad Q_1\qquad\qquad\quad P_{50}\qquad\qquad\qquad\quad Q_3$

The positions of the first quartile, the median and the third quartile have been indicated. Also, we have $\sum x = 141$ and $\sum x^2 = 1585.24$

(a) mean: $\bar{x} = \dfrac{\sum x}{n} = \dfrac{141}{14} = 10.07$

(b) median: half-way between 10.2 and 10.6, $P_{50} = 10.4$

(c) IQR: $IQR = Q_3 - Q_1 = 12.6 - 7.6 = 5$

(d) range: max − min = 15.4 − 5.0 = 10.4

EXAMPLE 3.4   cont.

(e) variance:
$$s^2 = \frac{\sum x^2 - \frac{(\sum x)^2}{n}}{n-1} = \frac{1585.24 - \frac{19881}{14}}{13}$$

$$s^2 = \frac{1585.24 - 1420.07}{13} = \frac{165.17}{13} = 12.71$$

(f) standard deviation: $s = \sqrt{s^2} = \sqrt{12.71} = 3.56$

Unbiased estimators

Most of the time we deal with samples, and our aim is to obtain some useful information which we can use to make inferences about the population from which the samples were taken. We have seen that dividing a sample sum of squares by the sample size n will lead to a *biased estimate* of the actual population variance. This bias is corrected by dividing by one less than the sample size, $n - 1$. This value, $n - 1$, is often referred to as the *number of degrees of freedom* associated with the sum of squares. Dividing by $n - 1$ for sample variances gives a better estimate of the population variance than would be obtained by dividing by n.

This can be readily seen from the Minitab simulation in Figure 3.5, which involved selecting 500 samples of size 20 from a defined *population* consisting of the integers 1 to 50. The variance for this population is $\sigma^2 = 208.2249$. Variances were calculated for each of the 500 samples in two ways. Those calculated by dividing $n - 1$ are labelled $Var(n - 1)$ and those calculated by dividing by n are labelled $Var(n)$. Notice that the average of the $Var(n - 1)$ variances is closer to the population variance of 208.2249 than the average of the $Var(n)$ variances. (Extra comments in the printout are in italics.)

This simulation suggests that, on average, the sample variance will give a consistently more accurate estimate of the true population variance if the sample sum of squares is divided by $n - 1$. This is not to say that any one particular sample will be more, or less, accurate than any other. We only have to look at the spread of the 500 sample variances in the Minitab printout above to see that some samples were considerably worse than others. And remember that *all* of the samples were taken from the same population, so each sample variance was in fact *estimating* the true population variance of 208.2249.

The coefficient of variation

The standard deviation may be used to compute a relative measure of dispersion called the coefficient of variation (CV). This statistic is useful for comparing the relative dispersion of distributions that have markedly different means, or different units of measurement. The coefficient of variation, like the standard deviation, is appropriate for quantitative variables and is reported with the mean.

The coefficient of variation is given by

$$CV = 100.\frac{s}{\bar{x}}$$

```
MTB > random 500 c1 - c20;
SUBC> integer 1 - 50.
MTB > rstdev c1 - c20 c21        Calculates sample standard deviations
MTB > let c22 = c21**2           Squaring to get sample variances
MTB > let c23 = c22*19/20        Converting to variances with 'n' in
                                 denominator
MTB > name c21 'Var(n-1)' c23 'Var(n)'
MTB > dotplot c22 c23;
SUBC> same.
```

```
The population variance (208.2249) is shown by the vertical dotted
line. Notice how the first dotplot is centred closer to this line
than the second. The table below shows that on average variances
calculated using n-1 in the denominator lie closer to the actual
population variance but are more spread.
```

```
MTB > desc c22 c23
```

	N	MEAN	MEDIAN	TRMEAN	STDEV	SEMEAN
Var(n-1)	500	205.83	206.49	206.02	39.46	1.76
Var(n)	500	195.54	196.17	195.72	37.48	1.68

	MIN	MAX	Q1	Q3
Var(n-1)	85.31	336.56	179.70	233.50
Var(n)	81.05	319.73	170.72	221.83

Figure 3.5 Minitab simulation of bias.

Practical statistics for the health sciences

3.6 Using Minitab to obtain descriptive statistics

Rather than relying upon the formulae for mean and variance, it is often much quicker and easier to use your calculator or a computer package like Minitab. The most useful command is DESCRIBE, which will print out all of the above statistics except the variance, which can be obtained simply by squaring the standard deviation. In the following Minitab printout the data concerning extra study hours per week was entered into column 1 and the basic descriptive statistics were obtained. Notice that the mean, median, and standard deviation can be obtained using separate commands if so desired. Again, input by the user is in bold type.

```
MTB > set c1
DATA> 11.6 10 11.4 12.6 7.6 7.8 5 5 10.2 5 10.6 14.2 14.6 15.4
DATA> end
MTB > name c1 'Study'

MTB > mean c1
  MEAN  =    10.071

MTB > median c1
  MEDIAN =    10.400

MTB > range c1
  RANGE  =    10.400

MTB > stdev c1
  ST.DEV. =    3.5644

MTB > desc c1


            N      MEAN    MEDIAN    TRMEAN    STDEV    SEMEAN
Study      14    10.071    10.400    10.050    3.564    0.953


           MIN      MAX      Q1       Q3
Study     5.000   15.400   6.950   13.000
```

Figure 3.6 Descriptive statistics from Minitab.

The specific commands for each of the individual summary statistics would need to be used if you wished to store the values of these statistics for use at some later stage. For example, the command MEAN c1 c2 calculates the mean for the data in column 1 and stores the result in column 2, wiping out any data that may have been in column 2. This very common trap is made worse by there being no warning from Minitab to inform you that you may be overwriting data. Similarly, the command LET K1 = STDEV c1 defines a constant, K1, to be the standard deviation of the data in column 1. Other statistics that are available from Minitab are median and range, as demonstrated in Figure 3.6. Minitab also has the facility to calculate means, medians and standard deviations of *rows of data* using the commands RMEANS, RMEDIANS and RSTDEV. The last of these commands was used in Figure 3.5 when simulating biased estimators.

3.7 Detecting outliers

Outliers — scores that differ so markedly from the main body of data as to raise questions concerning their accuracy — should be carefully examined. Their presence suggests the possibility of some form of data error or contamination. When collecting data there are many ways in which these errors can occur. Humans make mistakes — people misread instruments, transcribe numbers incorrectly, record data in the wrong place, present the wrong experimental conditions or instructions, and even fail to notice that equipment has malfunctioned. Machines do wear out, and may have faults.

It is not always possible to recognise these errors, as often they are data values that are indistinguishable from correct data and therefore go undetected. However, highly unusual scores will be easily spotted and should be checked. For example, the student nurse who described a patient as 17 m tall with a 3-week-old baby weighing 84 kg had definitely made data errors! Familiarity with the sample will help distinguish data errors from unusual observations.

3.8 Describing distributions

An initial investigation of a data set is usually referred to as *exploratory data analysis* (EDA) and is often characterised by a consideration of four aspects: shape, centre, spread and outliers.

(a) For quantitative data the *shape* of a distribution is important in that it gives us some idea of a possible model to use to represent the distribution. The shape may have one peak or several peaks, and it may appear to be balanced (ie symmetric) or perhaps skewed in one direction. Shape is irrelevant when dealing with categorical data.

(b) The *centre* of a distribution may be a particular value or a group of values, either individual or adjacent. Either way we are interested in where major clusters or groups of scores occur.

(c) The *spread* of a distribution focuses our attention on the range of values over which the distribution lies and how the values are spread, particularly with respect to the mean or the median.

(d) The presence of *outliers* in the data is always of interest because they may be errors, or gaps in the distribution. These will be scores that stand out from the rest of the data. Sometimes it is difficult to know whether to include or exclude these values in the analysis, particularly if they are not errors.

The worked example in Figure 3.7 is an investigation of the weights of a sample of 50 first-year students, comprising 30 males and 20 females. The weights were put into column 1 and the sex indicator (0 = female, 1 = male) was put into column 2.

```
MTB > print c1 c2

ROW   kg.    Sex 0 = female and 1 = male

  1  44.5455  0
  2  68.1818  1
  3  49.0909  0
  4  71.8182  1
  5  73.6364  1
  6  50.9091  0
  7  53.6364  0
  8  75.9091  1  Only the first eight values have been shown
                 here.

MTB > tally c2

   C2 COUNT
   0  20
   1  30
   N=  50            Checking to see that there are 20 females
                     and 30 males.

MTB > boxplot c1
```

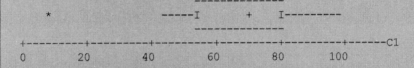

```
MTB > hist c1

Histogram of C1  N = 50
```

Both the boxplot above, and the histogram below confirm the presence of an outlier, which should be investigated further.

```
Midpoint  Count
   10      1 *
   20      0
   30      0
   40      1 *
   50     13 *************
   60      5 *****
   70     12 ************
   80     11 ***********
   90      6 ******
  100      1 *
```

In order to further investigate the outlier the data is printed and the values checked. The offending value has been highlighted in the printout below, and because it is impossible to have a weight of 8 kg the value has been excluded from the data set.

```
MTB > print c1

C1
 44.5455 68.1818 49.0909 71.8182 73.6364 50.9091 53.6364
 75.9091 77.2727 54.5455 80.4545 84.5455 86.8182 58.1818
 84.0909 88.6364 62.2727 93.1818 86.3636 54.5455 85.4545
 80.0000 53.6364 76.3636 52.2727 52.2727 73.6364 71.3636
 70.0000 67.2727 45.9091 65.0000 65.9091 49.0909 70.4545
 50.0000 70.0000 52.7273 73.1818 75.0000 64.5455 83.6364
 54.5455 77.2727 88.6364 60.0000 58.6364 97.7273  8.0000
 83.1818

MTB > delete 49 c1 c2

MTB > boxplot c1


              ---------------------
        ----------I        +        I------------------
              ---------------------
        ---------+---------+---------+---------+---------+---------C1
            50        60        70        80        90


MTB > hist c1


Histogram of C1  N = 49

Midpoint  Count
    45    2 **
    50    6 ******
    55    6 ******
    60    4 ****          Notice from the histogram that the
    65    4 ****          distribution seems to be bimodal.
    70    6 ******        There appear to be two main areas
    75    8 ********      of clumping, probably caused by
    80    2 **            combining the weights of males &
    85    7 *******       females.
    90    2 **
    95    1 *
   100    1 *

MTB > desc c1


           N      MEAN    MEDIAN    TRMEAN    STDEV    SEMEAN
C1        49     68.70     70.00     68.56    14.06     2.01

          MIN       MAX       Q1        Q3
C1      44.55     97.73    54.55     80.23
```

*Separate information can be obtained for males and females in this case because the sex indicators were placed into column 2. As males are generally heavier than females it makes sense to consider the data as separate cases. This is best achieved using the **by** subcommand in Minitab, as shown below.*

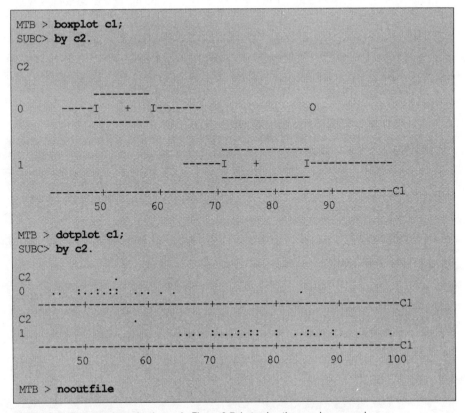

```
MTB > desc c1;
SUBC> by c2.

          C2    N      MEAN    MEDIAN   TRMEAN   STDEV   SEMEAN
C1        0    20     55.27    53.64    54.27    8.48    1.90
          1    29     77.96    76.36    77.71    8.52    1.58

          C2   MIN      MAX      Q1       Q3
C1        0    44.55   84.09    50.23    58.52
          1    65.00   97.73    70.91    85.00
```

Figure 3.7 Investigation of the weights of a sample of students: males vs females.

From the above summary it is clear that the males are heavier than the females.

Similar visual comparisons can be made using the **by** subcommand, and in fact we can see that the two groups are quite different. There is an outlier amongst the females which was not apparent from the combined data, and the distribution of male weights seems to be spread out more than the female weights, despite the similarity of their standard deviations. The outlier is exerting an influence here. The boxplots give an indication of the difference in the spread of the data in each case. The dotplots show the location of each data value, but do not give a very good indication of the shapes of the distributions because the samples were relatively small. Separate histograms would have been better for this purpose.

```
MTB > boxplot c1;
SUBC> by c2.

C2


0        -----I   +   I--------                    O



1                        ------I   +        I--------------

          --------+---------+---------+---------+---------+---------C1
              50        60        70        80        90

MTB > dotplot c1;
SUBC> by c2.

C2              .
0      ..  :..:.::   ... . .                         .
       -------+---------+---------+---------+---------+---------C1
C2              .
1                    ....  :...:.::  :  ..:.. :    .     .
       -------+---------+---------+---------+---------+---------C1
           50        60        70        80        90        100

MTB > nooutfile
```

Figure 3.8 The same investigation as in Figure 3.7, but using the BY subcommand.

Exercises

1 Let the variable x take the following values:
3, 2, 5, 3, 1
(a) $\Sigma x =$

(b) $\dfrac{\Sigma x}{n} =$

2 (a) What symbol is used for the mean of a population?
(b) What symbol is used for the mean of sample?

3 Give at least two reasons why the mean is such an important measure of central tendency.

4 Give two examples of situations where it would not be best to use the mean to describe the 'average' of a distribution.

5 (a) Find the mean, median and mode of the following scores:
2, 4, 3, 4, 4, 3, 1, 5, 4, 6
(b) What would happen to the mean, median and mode if the last score was increased by 7?
(c) If each observation were to be increased by 2, what effect would this have on the mean?

6 In a group of eight scores the mean is 4. If seven of the scores are:
6, 4, 3, 5, 2, 1, 6
what is the eighth score?

7 A patient's temperature was recorded hourly from 6 am to 6 pm. It was as follows:
36.8, 37.2, 37.9, 38.1, 38.2, 38.1, 38.2, 37.9, 37.6, 37.4, 37.1, 36.9
(a) What is the mean, median and mode of the recordings?
(b) Is this useful information to have? Why?
(c) When is it appropriate to use the mean, median or mode?

8 For each of the distributions in (a) to (d), state whether you would use the mean, mode, or median to represent the most appropriate central measure for each distribution.
(a) Failed at first attempt
(b) 1.2, 0.8, 1.1, .6, 25, 1.4
(c) 2, 3, 8, 5, 7, 8
(d) The annual income per Australian family.

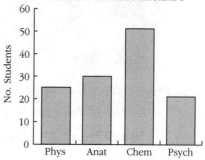

FAILED AT FIRST ATTEMPT

9 Draw a quick sketch to illustrate the probable shapes of each of the following four distributions.
(a) $\bar{x} = 56$; median = 62; mode = 68
(b) $\bar{x} = 68$; median = 62; mode = 56
(c) $\bar{x} = 62$; median = 62; mode = 62
(d) $\bar{x} = 62$; median = 62; mode = 30, 94

10 A sale of sports clothing was held in the Student Union building, The amounts (in dollars) spent by the first 20 customers were as follows:

53.80	98.50	29.30	42.20	28.40
79.00	30.00	28.50	35.70	5.90
42.00	35.00	37.50	85.00	76.50
91.20	45.25	54.60	65.65	72.85

What was the average amount spent by this group of students? What measure have you chosen and why? Would this value change if the outlier was removed?

11 A patient suffering from dementia was observed over nine 1-hour periods, and the number of times repeated questions were asked was recorded. The following data resulted:
24, 9, 12, 15, 10, 13, 22, 20, 14
Compute the following statistics for the data.
(a) mean
(b) median
(c) mode

12 The weight (kg) lost by 15 individuals who undertook a program of regular exercise (walking and cycling) for a 3-month period is listed below:
2.1 1.8 3.1 2.7 4.2 1.8 3.6 2.3
2.7 2.4 2.9 3.8 2.1 1.7 1.9
(a) Calculate the mean, median, and mode for

this data. Which measure best represents this data?

(b) Illustrate the data using a box-and-whisker plot.

13 The heights of 40 AFL footballers are listed below.

Collingwood				
193	183	178	191	189
189	192	178	170	194
185	173	184	183	180
203	185	170	193	183

Essendon				
191	189	175	188	183
181	188	183	178	192
190	179	206	186	172
198	185	178	198	183

(a) Calculate the mean, median and modal heights for each team and for the combined squad.

(b) Calculate the first and third quartiles for each group.

(c) Illustrate each height distribution using a box-and-whisker plot. (Use the same scale for each plot.)

14 Calculate n, Σx^2, and $(\Sigma x)^2$ for the following data sets:

(a) 2 1 1 3 4 6 2 1 3 1 4 8

(b) 30 17 12 20 17 17 30 30 15 12

(c) 10 10 20 20 20 30 30

15 For each data set above calculate
$n\Sigma x^2 - (\Sigma x)^2$

16 Which of the following data sets shows the greatest variability? Justify your choice.

(a)

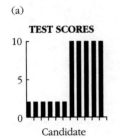

(b)

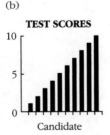

Calculate the range and standard deviation for each set of scores.

17 Indicate whether each of the following statements is True or False. If a statement is false, correct it by changing the wording.

(a) If the standard deviation of a distribution is large, the mean must be large also.

(b) In a symmetrical distribution the range is about 6σ.

(c) If the median of the distribution is known then the range will be the best index of spread to use.

(d) For a given distribution with $\mu = 0$, $\sigma = 1$, it is impossible to add two scores of different value to the distribution yet leave both μ and σ unchanged.

18 In a study of the efficiency of two different appointment systems, the waiting time (in minutes) before receiving attention was recorded for each client. The mean and standard deviation were reported.

	Room 1	Room 2
mean	60	50
standard deviation	10	100

Based on the above information, which system would you say is the most efficient?

19 The following figures are based on surveys conducted in Australia in 1990. Fifty male and fifty female smokers were asked how many cigarettes they usually smoke in one day. The results were as follows:

Males

1	11	25	27	8	7	5	4	25	12
6	12	6	18	25	4	15	13	21	30
6	15	17	5	22	30	3	14	35	35
15	25	25	16	26	45	13	50	25	34
13	12	15	24	24	45	15	30	26	17

Females

4	1	5	12	12	15	18	19	34	50
16	4	15	35	16	25	25	24	25	7
14	14	4	5	17	8	17	14	28	9
15	25	27	15	3	15	17	16	6	8
2	3	2	3	36	30	24	16	28	27

Use descriptive statistics to summarise this data and to compare male and female smoking habits.

20 In 1985 the numbers of Australians with suspected disc prolapse requiring surgery were as follows (Source: *Australian Family Physician*, Vol.14, No.11):

Age	Men	Women
0 – 14	18	6
15 – 24	233	197
25 – 34	946	473
35 – 44	1334	740
45 – 54	998	690
55 – 64	493	360
65+	233	290
Total	4255	2755

Describe this data: remember to mention the shape, centre and spread of the data.

Progress review 1

1 It is believed that hunger is partly controlled by external (environmental) cues. To investigate this a random sample of 60 first-year students was selected, and each student was randomly allocated to one of three groups. Each group of 20 students was put into a room with a large clock prominently displayed on the wall, and asked to complete a questionnaire. In the first room the clock on the wall showed the correct time. In the other rooms the clock was either one hour fast or one hour slow. The actual time, 5.30pm, was the usual evening meal time for all of the students. While the participants filled out the questionnaire, some dry biscuits and cheese were freely available. The weight of the biscuits and cheese consumed by each student was calculated; the means were: 4.30 group, 200 grams; 5.30 group, 300 grams; and 6.30 group, 400 grams.

For this study, identify:

(a) the dependent variable,
(b) the independent variable,
(c) a population of interest,
(d) a sample,
(e) a statistic that was calculated,
(f) a variable measured on a nominal scale, and
(g) a variable measured on a ratio scale.

Write a sentence that tells what the study found.

2 The following graph displays information obtained from a survey of 9500 Victorian Year 10 students taken in September 1992. The results of two previous surveys (in 1985 and 1989) are shown as 'Drugs used in the past'.

DRUG USE BY YEAR 10 STUDENTS

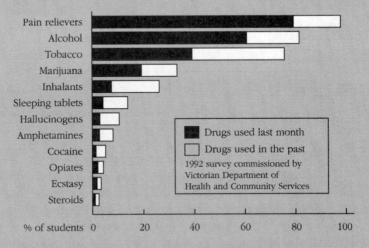

Source *The Age*, 5 March 1993

Use the graph to answer the following questions:

(a) Why was this type of graph used?
(b) Which drug was most commonly used last month?
(c) Which drug was most commonly used in the past?

(d) What proportion of students had smoked marijuana last month?

(e) How many students had taken alcohol in the past?

(f) (i) List the four most prevalent drugs that were used in the past.

(ii) How do they compare with the results of the September 1992 survey?

3 The following newspaper article makes three claims based on the data in the table:

Claim 1

The Bureau of Statistics figures show that the proportion of adult men employed has slumped more than three times as much as that of women.

Claim 2

For the first time, the male unemployment rate is now far higher than the female rate.

Claim 3

The male unemployment rate has more than doubled.

MEN: THE NEW UNEMPLOYED

	Trend employment levels		
	Jan 90 000	Jan 93 000	Change 000
MEN			
Employed full-time	4255	3896	-269
Employed part-time	370	450	80
Total in jobs	4625	4436	-189
% employed	71.2	65.2	-6.0
Unemployed	276	598	322
% unemployed	5.6	11.9	6.3
Not in labour force	1595	1773	178
WOMEN			
Employed full-time	1952	1903	-49
Employed part-time	1271	1346	75
Total in jobs	3224	3250	26
% employed	48.4	46.5	-1.9
Unemployed	232	372	140
% unemployed	6.7	10.3	3.6
Not in labour force	3211	3371	160

Source The Age. 13 February 1993, p3

(a) Using information from the table provided, determine whether each claim is justified.

(b) By how much did the number of men in work decline over the three-year period January 1990–January 1993?

(c) What was the corresponding change for the number of working women?

(d) The writer also claimed that the number of women unemployed jumped by 60%. How did he arrive at this value?

(e) The % unemployed is determined as follows:

$$\frac{\text{number unemployed}}{\text{total in jobs} + \text{number unemployed}} \times \frac{100}{1}$$

How were the % employed values determined?

4 (a) The following times (minutes) represent the length of telephone calls made by a sample of 15 students living on a college campus:

5, 4, 8, 7, 5, 4, 10, 6, 9, 5, 8, 4, 5, 5, 6

Calculate the following statistics for this data:

(i)   the median,

(ii) the interquartile range,

(iii) the mean,

(iv) the variance, and

(v)   describe the shape of the distribution.

(b) Use the following scores to answer the questions below:

−2, 4, 0, 1, 3, 6

Determine the following:

(i) $\sum x^2$,

(ii) $\sum(x + 2)$, and

(iii) the sum of the squared deviations of the scores from the mean.

5 The following numbers represent the scores of the top 10 golfers at a recent championship. Each of the 10 golfers had completed three rounds.

Scores

70	65	65	69	68	68	65	68	73	63	68	75
67	71	67	71	69	72	71	66	73	69	67	69
70	72	72	66	69	70

Use the Minitab printout below to answer the following questions:

(a) Describe the shape of the distribution.

(b) Use the histogram to determine the median and the mode.

(c) Determine the interquartile range.

(d) Draw a boxplot for this data.

```
MTB > hist c1

Histogram of score   N = 30

Midpoint  Count
   63     1 *
   64     0
   65     3 ***
   66     2 **
   67     3 ***
   68     4 ****
   69     5 *****
   70     3 ***
   71     3 ***
   72     3 ***
   73     2 **
   74     0
   75     1 *

MTB > desc c1

            N     MEAN   MEDIAN   TRMEAN    STDEV   SEMEAN
score      30   68.933      ?     68.923    2.803    0.512

            MIN      MAX      Q1       Q3
score    63.000   75.000   67.000   71.000

MTB > nooutfile
```

CHAPTER OUTLINE

CHAPTER FOUR

Probability

LEARNING OBJECTIVES

After studying this chapter, you should be able to:

- use conventional language to describe probability problems;
- use conventional mathematical notation to express probability problems;
- define and calculate the probability of a simple event;
- demonstrate an understanding of the fundamental mathematical concepts of probability, eg $0 \leq Pr(A) \leq 1$;
- distinguish between dependent and independent events;
- correctly identify mutually exclusive events;
- state the complement of a given event;
- list the events which would form collectively exhaustive outcomes of an experiment;
- correctly apply the addition and multiplication rules;
- recognise an example of conditional probability and correctly apply appropriate methods to solve these problems;
- use Venn diagrams to illustrate problems involving up to three events; and
- use contingency tables to clarify bivariate data and calculate their associated probabilities.

4.1   The nature of events

If you toss a coin into the air, most people would say that there is a 50% chance of it landing with heads facing up. Similarly, if you throw a six-sided die there is a 50% chance that an even number will result, or a one-in-six chance that any particular number, say two, will occur. These are examples of theoretical probabilities: probabilities that are worked out by considering the ratio of *favourable results to all possible results*. These are the probabilities that operate in many of the gambling games like Keno, Tattslotto and roulette.

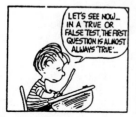 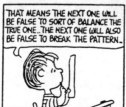 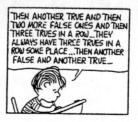 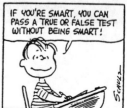

Source Linus: © 1952 United Features Syndicate, Inc. Reprinted by permission

On the other hand, tipping the winners of football matches or picking the winner of the Melbourne Cup generally involve what we call *subjective probabilities*. Probabilities of this type make use of *personal opinions* and *judgements* regarding what is likely to happen. For example, a fervent Adelaide supporter will have a different opinion regarding Adelaide's premiership chances than a serious Collingwood fan. These probabilities play an important part in everyday decision-making — when to invest in the share market, when to buy a new car, when to approach someone for a favour, and so on. Generally, we weigh up the situation by considering all possibilities, or relevant points, then we make a decision based upon the information at hand.

There are also probabilities derived from *empirical evidence*: that is, evidence that has been collected previously. We call these *empirical probabilities*, and examples can be found in the various premiums that are paid for house and car insurance, mortality tables, male/female births, and so on. Empirical probabilities are now being used more often in sport to determine the *likelihood* of certain results. For example, if Australia has won 18 of its past 20 cricket matches at the MCG, against England, then it seems reasonable to argue that they are highly likely to win their next match against England at the MCG.

If we are to make use of probabilities then we need to be able to *measure* them in some quantitative way. An impossible event is given a probability value of 0, while an event that is certain to occur is given a value of 1. All other probability values lie between 0 and 1. Providing that all possibilities are equally likely, the general definition for the probability of an event occurring is given by the following formula

$$\text{Pr(Event)} = \frac{\text{no. of favourable possibilities}}{\text{total no. of possibilities}}$$

The catch, of course, is to be able to determine the numerator and denominator of the fraction, as these may require considerable calculation. Knowledge of counting techniques such as permutations and combinations help.

Probability calculations need to take into account how the various events of interest are related to each other. These events can be categorised as independent, dependent, mutually exclusive, complementary or collectively exhaustive.

Independent events

Two events are independent if neither one is affected by the occurrence of the other. For example, when you roll a single die twice, the first result will have no effect upon the second result. The probability of getting a six on the second roll will be $\frac{1}{6}$, regardless of what was rolled first. Weekly Tattslotto draws are independent events because the numbers that 'came up' last week have no influence whatsoever on the numbers that will come up next week.

Dependent events

If the occurrence of the first event affects the probability of the second event occurring, then the second event is said to be *dependent* upon the first. For example, in a regular pack of cards the probability of drawing a second heart *after* a heart was initially drawn is $\frac{12}{51}$. The probability of wearing an overcoat before the weekend will depend upon the weather.

Mutually exclusive events

Two events are said to be mutually exclusive if they have no elements in common. This means that the occurrence of one event precludes the occurrence of the other. If a single card is drawn from a pack of cards, it is not possible for the drawn card to be a *heart* as well as being *black*. This is because the events classified as 'the card is a heart' and 'the card is black' are mutually exclusive. Similarly, it is not possible to get both 'a head' and 'a tail' in the one throw of a coin because the two events 'a head' and 'a tail', are mutually exclusive. It is possible, however, to get an odd number that is a three in a single throw of a die. The two events 'an odd number' and 'a three' are not mutually exclusive because they can both occur simultaneously.

Complementary events

The complement of an event consists of all outcomes in the sample space that are not part of the event. Hence the complement of the event 'the card is a heart' is the set of all cards that are not hearts. The probability of obtaining a heart is $\frac{13}{52}$, or $\frac{1}{4}$. The probability of not obtaining a heart is $\frac{39}{52}$, or $\frac{3}{4}$. Notice that if we add these two probabilities the result is 1. The following relationship between complementary events always holds:

$$\Pr(A) + \Pr(Not\ A) = 1$$

As another example, the probability of throwing a six is $\frac{1}{6}$, and the complementary probability, not throwing a six, is $\frac{5}{6}$. These two probabilities sum to 1. Often it is easier to calculate the probability of an event by first calculating the probability of its complement and then subtracting the result from one.

Collectively exhaustive events

A set of events in this category imply that no other event is possible in a given situation. For example, the three events 'the card is a heart', 'the card is a diamond' and 'the card is black' are collectively exhaustive because they exhaust all possibilities. In other words, all cards from a normal deck of playing cards can be put into one or the other of the nominated events.

EXAMPLE 4.1

Classify the following pairs of events according to whether they are
(a) independent or dependent;
(b) mutually exclusive;
(c) complementary;
(d) collectively exhaustive.
    (i)   Winning an Olympic gold medal / Setting a new Olympic record.
    (ii) Selecting a heart from a pack of cards / Selecting the king of spades (one draw only).
    (iii) Winning a prize in Keno this week / Winning a prize in Keno next week.
    (iv) Throwing an even number on a die / Throwing an odd number on a die.

Solution
(i)   Dependent, assuming that the gold medal and the Olympic record refer to the same event.
(ii) The two events are mutually exclusive.
(iii) Independent.
(iv) Independent, mutually exclusive, complementary and collectively exhaustive.

4.2   Rules of probability

In many applications we have to determine probabilities for combinations of events rather than for any particular event. For example, a potential sponsor of an Olympic athlete may well be interested in the chances of the athlete winning a gold medal at the next Olympic games. At the same time, they may also be interested in the chances of the athlete creating a new world record. Suppose we identify these two events (ie situations) as *Event A* and *Event B*. In some situations we may wish to find the probability that both events occur. That is, we wish to find the probability that the athlete will win gold *and* set a new world record at the same time. Using probability notation, we express this as *Pr(A and B)*. At other times we may wish to determine the probability that *either A or B* occurs. We denote this probability as *Pr(A or B)*. Note that the latter case requires some knowledge of the preceding case. To determine the probability of either A or B occurring, we need to know the probability of both occurring together, as well as the probabilities of each occurring separately. This is explained by the *addition rule*.

The addition rule — Pr(A or B)

The addition rule is used to compute the probability that either, or both, of two events will occur. This probability can be computed simply by considering those elements which satisfy Event A *plus* those satisfying Event B. From these we *subtract* any elements that are in common, ie elements belonging to both A and B, because these elements have already been considered when dealing with the two events separately. The formula describing this is

$$Pr(A \text{ or } B) = Pr(A) + Pr(B) - Pr(A \text{ and } B)$$

EXAMPLE 4.2

The personnel manager of a large hospital gathers information regarding the qualifications of all the nurses employed at the hospital. Of the 500 nurses employed, 270 have a university/college degree, 240 were hospital trained, and 100 were hospital trained but had done extra study to complete their degrees.

How many nurses were either hospital trained or university/college trained?
What is the probability of randomly selecting such a nurse for promotion?

Solution

We can use the addition rule mentioned above by letting Event A represent the hospital-trained nurses, and Event B represent those having a university/college degree. Then the number of nurses who were either hospital trained or had a university/college degree is given by:

$$n(A) + n(B) - n(A \text{ and } B) = 240 + 270 - 100 = 410$$

So, the probability of selecting such a nurse purely at random is 410/500, or 0.820. In other words, 82% of the nurses were either hospital trained or had a university/college degree. Note that the 100 nurses who satisfied both categories are subtracted because they are included in the Event A total as well as in the Event B total.

The situation described in the above example can be shown using a *Venn diagram*. Employees who have both types of degree are indicated by the *area of overlap* in the Venn diagram. This is shown in Figure 4.1, where the overlap has been shaded to provide extra emphasis. If 240 nurses have a university/college degree, and 100 of those were also hospital trained, it follows that 140 nurses have a university/college degree only. Similarly, we find that 170 nurses were hospital trained only. Therefore the number of nurses with either a university/college degree or hospital training, or both, can be expressed as: 140 + 170 + 100 = 410.

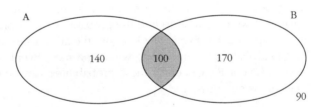

Figure 4.1 Venn diagram showing status of nurses.

The above Venn diagram also shows that 90 of the nursing staff employed had neither a university/college degree nor hospital training. This information was not immediately evident from the original data.

If the two events A and B are *mutually exclusive,* the shaded area would be empty because there would be no elements in common. This would mean that $\Pr(A \text{ and } B) = 0$, and therefore $\Pr(A \text{ or } B) = \Pr(A) + \Pr(B)$.

Conditional probability

Related events are dependent events; knowing that one has occurred is important for predicting the occurrence of the other. Knowing that a flower has not been watered will tell us something about the probability of it surviving. Knowing that an even number has occurred in a single throw of a fair die will tell us something about the probability that the number is a four. Knowing that an athlete has set new world records on each of the previous two occasions he has competed recently should tell us something about his chances of winning the event at a forthcoming athletics meet. These are examples of what we call *conditional probabilities*, where the probability of an event occurring depends upon the occurrence of some other event. In other words, we are interested in finding the probability of Event A occurring, given that Event B has already occurred. This is written as $Pr(A|B)$.

Consider Figure 4.1 again. Suppose a nurse is randomly chosen to be a staff representative at management meetings. Suppose we know that the employee selected was hospital trained (ie Event B has already occurred) and we now wish to compute the probability that the nurse also has a university/college degree (ie that Event A has occurred as well).

From the Venn diagram it can be seen that of the 270 nurses that were hospital trained, 100 also have a university/college degree. Therefore the probability of selecting a nurse with a university/college degree from those who have been hospital trained is $\frac{100}{270}$. Hence we have the *Conditional Probability Rule*, which states:

$$Pr(A|B) = \frac{Pr(A \text{ and } B)}{Pr(B)}$$

Conditional probabilities are not commutative; that is, $Pr(A|B) \neq Pr(B|A)$. This can be seen from Figure 4.1, where

$$Pr(B|A) = \frac{Pr(B \text{ and } A)}{Pr(A)}$$

You should note, however, that $Pr(A \text{ and } B) = Pr(B \text{ and } A)$.

The multiplication rule — Pr(*A* and *B*)

The *multiplication rule* is used to compute the probability that two events will both occur. The resulting probability is referred to as a *joint probability*. For example, we may wish to find the probability that a playing card is red (Event A), and is also an ace (Event B). Or, to use the athletics example, we may be interested in the probability of an athlete winning a race (Event A) and setting a new world record (Event B). Generally these probabilities can be determined using either of the following equations:

$$Pr(A \text{ and } B) = Pr(A).Pr(B|A) \quad \text{or} \quad Pr(B \text{ and } A) = Pr(B).Pr(A|B)$$

From Figure 4.1 we can see that 100 employees have both hospital training and a university/college degree. Therefore the probability of randomly selecting a nurse having both hospital training and a university/college degree is $\frac{100}{500}$, or 0.20. That is, $Pr(A \text{ and } B) = \frac{100}{500}$.

The Venn diagram can also be used to illustrate the multiplication rule. For example,

$$Pr(A) = \frac{240}{500}, Pr(B|A) = \frac{Pr(B \text{ and } A)}{Pr(A)} = \frac{100/500}{240/500} = \frac{100}{240}$$

$$\Pr(A \text{ and } B) = \Pr(A).\Pr(B|A) = \frac{240}{500} \cdot \frac{100}{240} = \frac{100}{500}$$

Now it becomes important to distinguish between *dependent* and *independent* events. The term 'independent' means not subject to bias or influence. If two events are independent, neither is affected by the occurrence of the other. If an influence is shown (ie dependency), then the probability of an event will change as information is obtained about the other event. This was seen in the conditional probability examples we looked at. If the probability of an event is not changed by additional knowledge about a second event, then the two events are independent. In this case we can state that $\Pr(A|B) = \Pr(A)$, and $\Pr(B|A) = \Pr(B)$. So, for two independent events we have the following rule:

$$\Pr(A \text{ and } B) = \Pr(A).\Pr(B)$$

Joint probabilities are often easiest to work out using *tree diagrams*, where the probabilities for individual events are represented by branches, as on a tree. Various combinations of events can then be determined by multiplying the respective probabilities. Consider, for example, a coin weighted in such a way that the probability of it landing heads is 0.60. Two throws of this coin can be represented by the tree diagram in Figure 4.2.

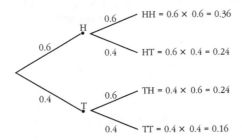

Figure 4.2 Tree diagram showing results of two throws of a biased coin. H = heads, T = tails.

EXAMPLE 4.3

Three people were needed to form a working party to investigate sexual harassment of students at a university campus. Fifty people, comprising 15 males and 35 females, expressed their interest in being a member of the working party. To form the working party it was decided to *randomly* choose three people from the 50 who expressed interest. Use a tree diagram to calculate the probability that the working party will consist of two males and one female.

Solution

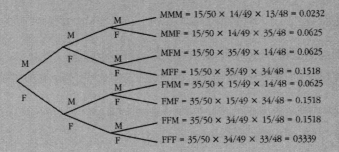

EXAMPLE 4.3 cont.

From the tree diagram, 2 males and 1 female resulted three times, each time with a probability of 0.0625. So the total probability of the working party consisting of 2 males and 1 female is $3 \times 0.0625 = 0.1875$.

Contingency tables

Sometimes information can be summarised in the form of a table, with the categories for one variable listed down one side and the categories for another variable listed across the top. Tables such as these are sometimes referred to as *contingency tables*. The information in the rows and columns of the table can be used to determine particular probabilities. The probability that an element selected at random will be in a particular category is found by dividing values in the table by the grand total.

Consider Table 4.1, which shows the number of patients in a surgical ward requiring observations. *Marginal* probabilities (the probabilities of one (or more) of the categories within either variable occurring) can be calculated by dividing the row totals by the grand total, or by dividing the column totals by the grand total. These represent the probabilities of (a) being a patient in either a public hospital or a private hospital, or (b) having an observation schedule that is 4-hourly or more, or one that is less than 4 hours.

Table 4.1 Surgical patients requiring observation, by hospital type.

Hospital	Observation schedule		Total
	≥ 4-hourly	< 4-hourly	
Public	14	6	20
Private	4	8	12
Total	18	14	32

For example, 20 of the 32 patients sampled were from public hospitals, so the probability of randomly selecting a public hospital patient from those sampled is $\frac{20}{32}$, or 0.6250. Similarly, the probability of randomly selecting a patient with an observation schedule that is less than 4 hours is $\frac{14}{32}$, or 0.4375.

Joint probabilities can also be worked out from the body of the table. Notice from the table that, of the 12 private hospital patients in the sample, 4 of them were on 4-hourly or more observation schedules. The probability of randomly selecting a private hospital patient who was on a 4-hourly or more observation schedule is a joint probability, and is read from the table as $\frac{4}{32}$, or 0.1250. This can be verified by using the general rule for finding joint probabilities, ie $\Pr(A \text{ and } B) = \Pr(A).\Pr(B|A)$. If we define the random selection of a private hospital patient as A and the selection of a patient on a 4-hourly or more observation schedule as B, then we have the following:

$$\Pr(A) = \tfrac{12}{32} \qquad \text{and} \qquad \Pr(B|A) = \tfrac{4}{32}$$

therefore $\Pr(A \text{ and } B) = \tfrac{12}{32} \times \tfrac{4}{12} = \tfrac{4}{32}$

Notice the ease of determining the conditional probability $Pr(B|A)$. Given that there were 12 private hospital patients in the sample, and 4 of them on a 4-hourly or more observation schedule, the conditional probability of $\frac{4}{12}$ follows.

EXAMPLE 4.4

A random sample of 90 male and 60 female students was asked to indicate a major area of interest with respect to the courses they were studying. The results were summarised as follows:

Thirty per cent of the total sample indicated that psychology was of major interest. Half of the females were mainly interested in sociological issues, whilst sports medicine was chosen by 50 males and 10 females. All students indicated one of the abovementioned areas of interest.

Summarise the information above in the form of a contingency table and use the table to determine the probabilities of:
(a) randomly selecting a female student from the sample;
(b) randomly selecting a student interested in sociological issues;
(c) randomly selecting a male interested in psychology.

Solution
The contingency table is as follows:

Interest	Male	Female	Total
Psychology	25	20	**45**
Sociology	15	**30**	45
Sports Medicine	**50**	**10**	60
Total	**90**	**60**	**150**

The bold numbers were given in the initial summary. These were put into the table first of all, thus enabling the remainder of the table to be filled in.

(a) The probability of randomly selecting a female student is $\frac{60}{150} = 0.40$.

(b) The probability of randomly selecting a student interested in sociological issues is $\frac{45}{150} = 0.30$.

(c) The probability of randomly selecting a male interested in psychology is $\frac{25}{150} = 0.1667$.

1 Classify the following events as independent or dependent:
  (a) a cloudy sky and rain,
  (b) tossing a head and rolling a 6,
  (c) dealing a king, then an ace, without replacement,
  (d) choosing a king, replacing that card then choosing an ace.

2 Give two examples of mutually exclusive events.

3 Give two examples of exhaustive events.

4 When a single die is rolled there are six possible outcomes.
  (a) List the outcomes comprising each of the following events:
    A = the event the die comes up even,
    B = the event the die comes up four or more,
    C = the event the die comes up at most two,
    D = the event the die comes up three.
  (b) Calculate the following probabilities:
    (i) $\Pr(A)$; (ii) $\Pr(A \text{ or } B)$; (iii) $\Pr(A \text{ and } B)$; (iv) $\Pr(C)$; (v) $\Pr(C \text{ and } D)$; (vi) $\Pr(C \mid A)$

5 One hundred physical education students were surveyed to determine what injuries they had suffered in the past six months. It was found that 20 had suffered arm injuries, 30 leg injuries and 60 had suffered neither. Five had suffered head injuries, but none of these had suffered arm or leg injuries. Use a Venn diagram to determine the probability of randomly selecting a student who had suffered:
  (a) an arm injury only,
  (b) a leg injury only,
  (c) an arm and a leg injury,
  (d) an arm or a leg injury,
  (e) no injury.

6 At a certain university, 90% of first-year Humanities students are enrolled in English, 80% are enrolled in Psychology and 75% are enrolled in both courses. A student is randomly selected. Find the probability that the student is:

  (a) not enrolled in English,
  (b) enrolled in either English or Psychology,
  (c) enrolled in English given that the student is enrolled in Psychology.

7 An experiment consists of flipping an unbiased coin until a head occurs, using a maximum of three tosses.
  (a) Using a tree diagram, list the sample space for this experiment and assign the appropriate probabilities to each sample point.
  Suppose the event H is defined as 'a head occurred' and event T as 'three tosses were required'.
  (b) Are H and T mutually exclusive events? Explain.
  (c) Are H and T independent events? Explain.

8 Let M = the event of having a son,
    L = the event of having a left-handed child,
    C = the event of being colour-blind.
  Assume the probability of having a son is $\frac{1}{2}$, the probability of being left-handed is $\frac{1}{5}$ and the fraction of colour-blind males is $\frac{1}{12}$.
    Assume also that handedness is independent of gender. Calculate the following probabilities, stating any further assumptions you feel you may need to make:
  (a) having a left-handed son,
  (b) having a colour-blind son,
  (c) having a left-handed but not colour-blind son.

9 After extensive investigation the probability distribution of coloured lollies in packets of a particular brand was found to be as follows:

Colour	Probability
Brown	0.3
Red	0.2
Yellow	?
Green	0.1
Orange	0.1
Tan	0.1

On the basis of this information, what is the probability of selecting a yellow lolly? Why?

10 Use the information in Question 9 to find the probability of each of the following events:

(a) you select a brown or red lolly,

(b) you select a green, red or tan lolly,

(c) the lolly you draw is not yellow,

(d) the lolly you draw is neither orange nor tan,

(e) you select a brown, red, yellow, green, orange or tan lolly.

11 A survey is taken of 150 residents of a small resort town to determine attitudes of the residents towards a proposed hotel development. The occupations of the residents were determined, along with whether or not they approved of the hotel being built.

Attitude	Building and trade	Business	Other
Approve	40	40	5
Disapprove	10	20	35

Find the proportion of the 150 residents that:

(a) are business people,

(b) approve of the hotel being built,

(c) approve of the hotel being built, given that they are in building and trade,

(d) are business people given that they approve of the development being built, and

(e) are business people or approve of the development being built.

(f) Are events 'business people' and 'approve' independent? Are they mutually exclusive? Explain your answers.

12 The age and preferred area of employment of 7641 persons registered as unemployed in a provincial city in December 1991 were as follows:

Prefer	15–17	18–19	20–24	25–44
Admin	0	5	44	71
Profes	2	33	211	203
Art/Sport	5	11	24	40
Clerical	265	672	949	1259
Agricult	24	23	46	110
Manufact	122	204	288	708
Transport	5	14	72	367
Manual	92	168	563	1036
Other	0	0	2	3

An unemployed person is selected at random from this group, determine the probability that this person is:

(a) Seeking employment in manufacturing?

(b) Aged between 20–24 years.

(c) Aged between 20–24 years and seeking employment in manufacturing.

(d) Aged between 20–24 given that he/she is seeking employment in manufacturing.

(e) Seeking employment in manufacturing given that he/she is aged between 20–24.

CHAPTER OUTLINE

CHAPTER FIVE

Discrete probability distributions

LEARNING OBJECTIVES

After reading this chapter, you should be able to:
- list all possible outcomes of a simple experiment and their associated probabilities, thus forming a discrete probability distribution;
- calculate the expected value and variance for a discrete probability distribution;
- calculate the mean and variance for sums and differences of two independent random variables;
- recognise situations for which a binomial or Poisson distribution is an appropriate model;
- use formulae, statistical tables or Minitab to calculate binomial and Poisson probabilities;
- calculate the mean and variance for a binomial distribution;
- calculate the mean and variance of a Poisson distribution; and
- recognise when the binomial distribution may be approximated by the Poisson distribution.

5.1   *What is a probability distribution?*

The midwifery ward of a small country hospital has four cribs available for use at any time for newborn babies. From historical records kept by the hospital it can be shown that the probabilities of there being 0, 1, 2, 3 or 4 or more births in any one week are respectively 0.92, 0.04, 0.02, 0.01 and 0.01. We can define a random variable X to be the number of births at the hospital in any given week, and thereby summarise the situation as follows:

Number of births $(X = x)$	Probability $(X = x)$
0	0.92
1	0.04
2	0.02
3	0.01
$\geqslant 4$	0.01

This model is an example of a probability distribution. A probability distribution consists of a list of all of the possible values that a random variable X can take, together with the probabilities of those values occurring. These probabilities will add to one because the list of possibilities is mutually exclusive and exhaustive. In some ways probability distributions are similar to frequency distributions in that each associates a number with possible values assumed by a variable. A frequency distribution always describes a set of data that has actually been observed: that is, it is empirical. A probability distribution *may* be empirical, but it can *also* describe data that you could expect to observe under certain well-specified conditions. Hence, probability distributions may be hypothetical, or theoretical. Hypothetical or theoretical probability distributions can be found for games of chance involving dice, cards, lotto games, and so on. Empirical distributions can be found in quality control, the insurance industry, medical illness, sports results and many other areas. Personal decisions as to whether or not a particular horse or team will win an event may be influenced by previous performances (empirical) or may simply be based upon a whim (subjective).

Probability distributions are used in inferential statistics as models of how random variables are *expected* to behave. If the empirical data deviates appreciably from the predictions of a model, doubt is cast upon the correctness of the model or its assumptions. For example, the odds of selecting the joker from a pack of cards is 1 in 53 if the cards are well shuffled. If a card player can select the joker five times in a row, with the cards shuffled each time, then one might suspect that the cards had been marked in some way. The game would not seem to be fair.

Random variables may be discrete or continuous. For example the number of babies delivered last week is a discrete random variable because it can only assume integer values (0, 1, 2, 3, etc.). However, the lengths and weights of the babies are examples of continuous random variables, as an infinite number of lengths and weights are possible. Measurements on continuous random variables are usually restricted, however, by the accuracy of the measuring instruments. Birth weights, for example, are usually measured to the nearest gram.

5.2   *Discrete probability distributions*

Discrete probability distributions form an important part of our everyday lives. For example, consider the case where organisers of an outdoor concert wish to hold the event over a three-day weekend in a locality where there is a 50% chance of rain on any given day of the year. What weather outcomes are possible (ie fine or wet), and what are the respective probabilities associated with each of these possibilities? The tree diagram below outlines each possibility and also enables the respective probabilities to be calculated. We know that the chances of wet weather (W) are the same as that for fine weather (F), ie $\Pr(W) = 0.5 = \Pr(F)$, and we will assume that independence applies.

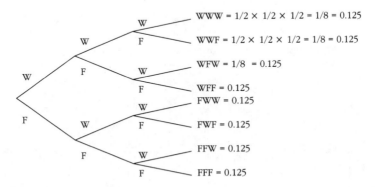

From the tree diagram you can see, for example, that there are three ways in which there could be one wet day and two fine days:

      (a) WFF — a wet day followed by two fine days; P = 0.125

      (b) FWF — a fine day, followed by a wet day, then a fine day; P = 0.125

      (c) FFW — two fine days, followed by a wet day; P = 0.125

Each of these combinations results in one wet day and two fine days. Therefore the probability of there being one wet day over the three-day weekend is found by summing the three probabilities: $\Pr(1W, 2F) = 0.125 + 0.125 + 0.125 = 0.375$. Now we can summarise all possibilities for the weather for the weekend in the form of a table. Table 5.1 represents the probability distribution for the random variable *the number of wet days over a three-day weekend*.

Table 5.1 Probability distribution for the number of wet days over a three-day weekend.

No. of wet days	Probability
0	0.125
1	0.125 + 0.125 + 0.125 = 0.375
2	0.125 + 0.125 + 0.125 = 0.375
3	0.125

Notice that there are four possibilities: zero, one, two, or three wet days, and that these possibilities are exactly the same as three, two, one, or zero fine days. Notice also that the probabilities sum to one; this is a feature of all probability distributions.

EXAMPLE 5.1

Two fair dice are rolled and the sum of their upturned faces is noted. Determine the probability distribution for the sum of the upturned faces, and use the results to find the probability that the sum in any one throw is greater than 5 but less than 10. Also find the sum that is most likely to occur.

Solution

First, list the possible combinations for the two dice.

1,1	1,2	1,3	1,4	1,5	1,6	2,1	2,2	2,3	2,4	2,5	2,6
3,1	3,2	3,3	3,4	3,5	3,6	4,1	4,2	4,3	4,4	4,5	4,6
5,1	5,2	5,3	5,4	5,5	5,6	6,1	6,2	6,3	6,4	6,5	6,6

We assume that each of the 36 possibilities is equally likely to occur, and we let X be the sum of the two dice and $Pr(X)$ be the probability of each sum occurring. The above possibilities produce the following table, with sums ranging from 2 to 12.

X	$Pr(X)$
2	1/36
3	2/36
4	3/36
5	4/36
6	5/36
7	6/36
8	5/36
9	4/36
10	3/36
11	2/36
12	1/36

(a) We want the sum greater than 5 but less than 10; ie $Pr(5 < X < 10)$.

Now $Pr(5 < X < 10) = Pr(X = 6, 7, 8 \text{ or } 9)$

$$= \frac{5}{36} + \frac{6}{36} + \frac{5}{36} + \frac{4}{36}$$

$$= \frac{20}{36} = 0.5556$$

(b) The most likely sum to occur is that which has the highest chance of occurring. $Pr(X = 7)$ has the highest probability of occurring (ie $\frac{6}{36}$), therefore it is the most likely result from a single throw of two fair dice.

Expected values (means)

We calculate averages for probability distributions in much the same way as we do for frequency distributions. For example, if we wish to calculate the average sum we would expect to score when rolling two dice over a long period of time, we multiply each possible sum by its respective probability and simply add the results. This is the same as calculating a weighted mean, because some of the sums occur more frequently than others. A sum equal to 7 can occur in six ways whereas a sum equal to 10 can occur in only three ways. The probabilities (relative frequencies) are used as the weightings, so the expected value (mean) of a discrete probability distribution is defined as follows:

$$E(X) = \sum x.\Pr(X = x)$$

The expected value for the sum of two dice is therefore

$$E(X) = \sum x.\Pr(X = x) = 2(\tfrac{1}{36}) + 3(\tfrac{2}{36}) + 4(\tfrac{3}{36}) + \ldots + 12(\tfrac{1}{36})$$

$$= \tfrac{2}{36} + \tfrac{6}{36} + \tfrac{12}{36} + \ldots + \tfrac{12}{36}$$

$$= \tfrac{252}{36}$$

$$= 7$$

In this case the expected value is the same as the value that is most likely to occur. This is not always so because not all discrete probability distributions are symmetrical about their midpoint. In some cases the expected value may not even be a value that the random variable can assume (see Example 5.2). Some care is needed in interpreting such cases: it is not possible for one couple to have 1.5 boys, but it is possible for two couples to have three boys.

EXAMPLE 5.2

Consider a couple who wish to have three children. How many boys can they expect to have, assuming that there is an equal chance of having either a boy or a girl?

Solution
The probability distribution table is:

No. of boys	Probability
0	0.125
1	0.375
2	0.375
3	0.125

$$E(X) = 0(0.125) + 1(0.375) + 2(0.375) + 3(0.125)$$
$$= 0.375 + 0.750 + 0.375$$
$$= 1.5$$

Variance of a probability distribution

In Chapter 3 we defined the variance as

$$\sigma^2 = \frac{\sum (x - \mu)^2}{N}$$

This, in turn, can be shown to be

$$\frac{\sum x^2 - N\mu^2}{N} = \frac{\sum x^2}{N} - \mu^2$$

The first term of the last expression is the *average* of the x^2 values. Therefore we can define the variance as

$$\text{Var}(X) = E[X - E(X)]^2 = E(X^2) - [E(X)]^2$$

The standard deviation is the square root of the variance and is given as

$$\text{St.Dev.}(X) = \sqrt{\text{Var}(X)} = \sqrt{E(X^2) - [E(X)]^2}$$

Calculating the variance is often long and tedious, and its interpretation is not as straightforward as that for the expected value. The variance is probably best thought of as a *squared* amount by which a random variable can be expected to deviate from its average, or expected value, over a long period of time. In order to calculate the variance, two quantities are required: $E(X)$ and $E(X^2)$. The latter is defined as $E(X^2) = \sum x^2 \Pr(X = x)$.

EXAMPLE 5.3

Determine the variance for the distribution of boys in a family of three children, assuming that the chances of having either a boy or a girl are the same.

Solution
First we have the probability distribution from Example 5.2:

No. of boys	Probability
0	0.125
1	0.375
2	0.375
3	0.125

Also, from Example 5.2 we know that $E(X) = 1.5$. We need to find $E(X^2)$.
$E(X^2) = \sum x^2 . \Pr(X = x) = 0^2(0.125) + 1^2(0.375) + 2^2(0.375) + 3^2(0.125)$
$E(X^2) = 0 + 0.375 + 4(0.375) + 9(0.125) = 0.375 + 1.5 + 1.125 = 3$

Now we can calculate the variance using the definition above.
$\quad \text{Var}(X) = E(X^2) - [E(X)]^2 = 3 - (1.5)^2 = 3 - 2.25 = 0.75$

The standard deviation is the square root of the variance, which in this case is
$\text{St.Dev}(X) = \sqrt{\text{Var}(X)} = \sqrt{0.75} = 0.867$

Mean and variance of two independent random variables

Imagine having to prepare a meal comprising spaghetti and a meat sauce, and being restricted to a one-element stove. The question of interest is: How long would you expect to take to prepare the meal? This is an example of finding the expected value for the sum of two independent random variables. We can define the random variable X to be the time taken to prepare the meat sauce, and Y to be the time taken to prepare the spaghetti. If on average it takes 20 minutes to prepare the meat sauce and 8 minutes to prepare the spaghetti, it seems reasonable to assume that the average time taken to prepare the complete meal would be the sum of the averages for each component of the meal. This is shown algebraically as follows:

$$E(X + Y) = E(X) + E(Y)$$

Similarly, we may be interested in the *differences* in times taken to prepare each of the components of the meal, and in particular we may want to know what the average difference in their times is likely to be. This is an example of an expected value for the difference between two independent random variables, and is defined as

$$E(X - Y) = E(X) - E(Y)$$

Regardless of whether we are interested in the sum or the difference of two independent random variables, the variation of each random variable will contribute to the overall variation of both the sum and the difference. If we combine the preparation times for both components of the meal, the resulting variation in the combined times will be due to the variation of each individual component. In other words

$$Var(X + Y) = Var(X) + Var(Y)$$

Although it might seem strange, the same argument applies for the variation in the differences between two independent random variables. The time taken to prepare the meat sauce will have a particular variation, and so too will the time taken to prepare the spaghetti. Whether we combine their times, or find the difference between their times, is irrelevant with regard to the overall variation. Variation in the differences between their times will still be made up of the variation in the times taken to prepare each part of the meal. So we have

$$Var(X - Y) = Var(X) + Var(Y)$$

Remember that this applies only to two independent random variables. If the random variables are not independent, one will have some influence over the other and this usually leads to some degree of interaction between the two variables. This interaction can be measured by what is defined to be the *covariance* of the variables, $Cov(X, Y)$.

EXAMPLE **5.4**

A component of an aerobic fitness machine consists of a metal disc fixed to the end of a cylindrical rod. The parts are made separately and then welded together as shown.

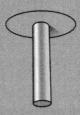

The metal disc has an average thickness of 1.5 cm and variance of 0.1 cm. The rod has an average length of 9 cm with a variance of 0.2 cm.

Find the expected value and the variance for the overall height of the component. (Ignore the thickness of the weld.)

EXAMPLE **5.4**   **cont.**

Solution

Define X to be the thickness of the metal disc and Y to be the length of the cylindrical rod. We then require $E(X + Y)$, and $Var(X + Y)$.

$$E(X + Y) = E(X) + E(Y) = 1.5 + 9 = 10.5 \text{ cm}$$
$$Var(X + Y) = Var(X) + Var(Y) = 0.1 + 0.2 = 0.3 \text{ cm}$$

We can expect the assembled component to have an average height of 10.5 cm with a variance of 0.3 cm.

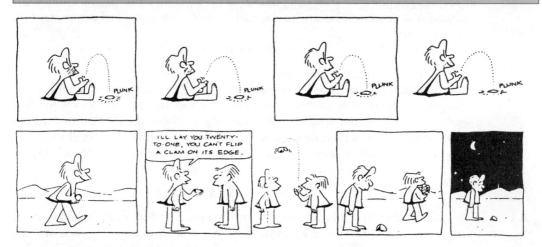

Source © Creators Syndicate International

5.3   *The binomial distribution*

In our electronically aware age we frequently encounter situations where only two possible results can occur. For example, a television is turned either on or off, the video has either recorded the film or it has not, the microwave is on or off. In fact, any switch is either on or off, because the electricity goes through the circuit or it doesn't. Non-mechanical problems may be viewed in the same way: a patient may either live or die, a bone may either be fractured or not, a new baby is either a boy or a girl, and a coin tossed into the air will land either heads or tails. Each of these situations can be represented by a discrete random variable that can assume only two states. Situations like this are often called *Bernoulli experiments* or Bernoulli trials. Our interest is usually in the outcome of several Bernoulli trials: tossing a coin n times and noting the number of heads, or randomly sampling n students and counting the smokers.

Many real-life situations or experiments can be set up so they have only two possible outcomes. Using probability jargon, these outcomes can be called *success* and *failure*. A new drug is effective or it is not; a patient is given the correct dosage or an incorrect dosage; a job is given to an applicant or it is not. These kinds of experimental situations can be modelled by the binomial distribution, enabling us to calculate the probabilities associated with the outcomes of repeated Bernoulli trials.

Consider a young couple wanting to start a family. Both parents might prefer to have a baby girl as their first child, so we could define the birth of a baby girl as a success for this couple. We will assume the probability of this to be 0.49. Now we consider this scenario in the light of more formal probability language.

The probability of observing a success (baby girl) on any given trial (birth) is denoted by p ($p = 0.49$) and the probability of failure (baby boy), by $1 - p$ or q ($q = 0.51$). Since the two outcomes, success and failure, are mutually exclusive (baby is either a boy or a girl) and exhaustive (no other possibilities), $p + q = 1$. When there are n Bernoulli trials (births), the random variable of interest is x, the number of successes (how many girls). The minimum number of successes is zero, while the maximum will be n.

The characteristics of a Bernoulli trial are as follows:

- a trial can result in one of two outcomes;
- the probability of a success remains constant from trial to trial; and
- the outcomes of successive trials are independent.

It is difficult for real-life situations to satisfy these requirements perfectly. The last two characteristics are satisfied only when sampling is done with replacement or from a sufficiently large (infinite) population, which is often not the case with most research sampling. However this practical departure from the ideal is of little consequence as long as the population is large relative to the sample size.

What if the same young couple wanted a family of four girls? We let the birth of a girl denote 'success', so therefore the birth of a boy would denote a 'failure'. Here $p = $ Pr(success) $= 0.49$ and $q = 1 - p = 0.51$. Also, we let X represent the number of successes (ie the number of girls), so X may take the values 0, 1, 2, 3 or 4. Table 5.2 summarises the situation by listing all possible results together with a summary of the number of baby girls occurring and the associated probabilities.

Table 5.2 Probability table of the results of four births.

Birth				No. of girls X	No. of combinations	$Pr(X = x)$
1	2	3	4			
G	G	G	G	4	1	$0.49^4 = 0.0576$
B	G	G	G			
G	B	G	G	3	4	$4(0.49)^3 0.51$
G	G	B	G			$= 0.2400$
G	G	G	B			
B	B	G	G			
B	G	B	G			
B	G	G	B	2	6	$6(0.49)^2(0.51)^2$
G	B	B	G			$= 0.3747$
G	B	G	B			
G	G	B	B			
B	B	B	G			
B	B	G	B	1	4	$4(0.49)(0.51)^3$
B	G	B	B			$= 0.2600$
G	B	B	B			
B	B	B	B	0	1	$0.51^4 = 0.0677$
Total possibilities = 16						$\Sigma p = 1.0$

The following worked example makes use of the results from the table above in relation to the number of girls in a family of four children. We are assuming here that the birth of children satisfies the characteristics of repeated Bernoulli trials.

EXAMPLE 5.5

Use the results from Table 5.2 above to find the probabilities of obtaining the following numbers of girls in families of four children, given that the probability of having a girl is 0.49:
(a) two girls, (b) three or more girls, (c) at least two girls, (d) no more than one girl.

Solution
(a) $\Pr(X = 2) = 0.3747$
(b) $\Pr(X \geq 3) = \Pr(X = 3 \text{ or } 4) = 0.2400 + 0.0576 = 0.2976$
(c) $\Pr(X \geq 2) = \Pr(X = 2, 3 \text{ or } 4) = 0.3747 + 0.2400 + 0.0576 = 0.6723$
(d) $\Pr(X \leq 1) = \Pr(X = 0 \text{ or } 1) = 0.0677 + 0.2600 = 0.3277$

While tables like Table 5.2 can be used to calculate probabilities rather than working from first principles, they soon get tedious for large values of n. Imagine the effort involved in analysing 20 births (not that a family would consider having 20 children these days!). It turns out that the coefficients of the expansion $(p + q)^4$ are the same as those values that occur in the column headed 'No. of combinations' in Table 5.2. Expanding $(p + q)^4$ we get the following:

$$(p + q)^4 = 1.p^4 + 4.p^3q + 6.p^2q^2 + 4.pq^3 + 1.q^4$$

If we substitute the appropriate values for p and q into the above equation then we get the probabilities associated with the number of successes, as they appear in the final column of Table 5.2. For $p = 0.49$ and $q = 0.51$,

$$(p + q) = 1(0.49)^4 + 4(0.49)^3(0.51) + 6(0.49)^2(0.51)^2 + 4(0.49)(0.51)^3 + 1(0.51)^4$$
$$= 0.0576 + 0.2400 + 0.3747 + 0.2600 + 0.0677$$

Notice that these values are the same as those in the $\Pr(X = x)$ column of Table 5.2. The number of successes in a series of repeated Bernoulli trials is called a *binomial random variable,* and the associated probability distribution is called the *binomial distribution*. Binomial probabilities are determined by four pieces of information:

(i) the number of trials, n;
(ii) the number of successes, x;
(iii) the probability of a success, p;
(iv) the number of ways in which x successes can be achieved.

The coefficients in the expansion of $(p + q)^4$ simply represent the number of ways in which the specified number of successes can be achieved. For example, three successes (ie three girls) can be achieved in four ways, and these are listed in Table 5.2. Rather than listing all the possible combinations, which is very tedious for large values of n, it is often easier to use the formula

$$^nC_x = \frac{n!}{x!(n - x)!}$$

For $n = 4$ and $x = 3$, $n! = 4 \times 3 \times 2 \times 1 = 24$, $x! = 3 \times 2 \times 1 = 6$ and $(n - x)! = 1! = 1$, so ${}^nC_x = {}^4C_3 = \dfrac{24}{6 \times 1} = 4$ ways of getting 3 successes in 4 trials.

Theoretical binomial probabilities can be calculated using the binomial formula. This formula gives the probability of x successes in n trials, assuming the probability of a success to be p. It is stated as follows:

$$\Pr(x) = {}^nC_x\, p^x (1 - p)^{n-x}$$

Fortunately, tables have been developed to help compute probabilities resulting from binomial distributions. To make use of these tables you need to know the values for n, for x, and for p. Most sets of tables do not go beyond $n = 20$, and often only have values for p in multiples of 0.10 or 0.05.

EXAMPLE 5.6

Using a set of binomial tables, determine:
(a) the probability of getting exactly 6 heads from 12 tosses of a fair coin,
(b) the probability of getting at most 4 heads from 15 tosses of a fair coin,
(c) in a multiple choice test of 10 questions, with each question having 4 choices, find the probability of passing (ie 50% or more) if the answer to each question is chosen by guessing.

Solution
For each case determine values for n, x and p.
(a) $n = 12$, $x = 6$, $p = 0.5$. From the tables we get $\Pr(x = 6) = 0.2256$.
(b) $n = 15$, $x = 0, 1, 2, 3,$ or 4, $p = 0.5$. From the tables we get
   $\Pr(x \le 4) = 0.0000 + 0.0005 + 0.0032 + 0.0139 + 0.0417 = 0.0592$.
(c) $n = 10$, $x = 5, 6, 7, 8, 9,$ or 10, $p = 0.25$. From the tables we get
   $\Pr(x \ge 5) = 0.0584 + 0.0162 + 0.0031 + 0.0004 + 0.0000 + 0.0000$
   $= 0.0781$.

You can use Minitab to calculate binomial probabilities more quickly and easily than either the tables or the binomial formula. The advantage of using a program like Minitab is that you are not limited in the values of n or p. This is particularly useful for values of p that are not contained in the tables. The printout below shows the theoretical binomial probabilities for $n = 6$ and $p = 0.375$ (ie. $p = \frac{3}{8}$). As can be seen from this printout the probability of 3 successes is 0.2575. Most tables would not have a p-value of 0.375, and to use the formula is a little tedious. Notice that with the **pdf** command in Minitab, values for n and p must be specified with the subcommand **binomial**.

```
MTB > pdf;
SUBC> binomial n=6, p=0.375.

 BINOMIAL WITH N =  6 P = 0.375000
  K       P( X = K)
  0       0.0596
  1       0.2146
  2       0.3219
  3       0.2575
  4       0.1159
  5       0.0278
  6       0.0028
MTB > nooutfile
```

By plotting the probabilities on a vertical axis and the values for the random variable X on the horizontal axis, graphs of these distributions can be drawn to emphasise their symmetry or skewness. The figure below shows a series of binomial distributions with $n = 4$, and various values for p. The graphs show that a binomial distribution will be symmetrical for $p = 0.50$, skewed to the right for $p < 0.50$, and skewed to the left when $p > 0.50$.

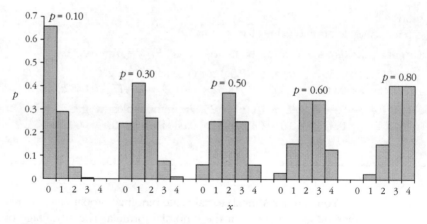

Figure 5.1 Histograms of various binomial distributions for n = 4.

The mean and variance of a binomial distribution

The binomial distribution is a discrete probability distribution, and it has a mean and a variance. The mean of a binomial distribution is the long-run average (the expected value) of a binomial random variable, and the variance is a measure of variation from this expected value. For example, consider the binomial distribution with $n = 4$ and $p = 0.5$.

X	0	1	2	3	4
$\Pr(X=x)$	0.0625	0.2500	0.3750	0.2500	0.0625

The expected value and the variance are:

$$E(X) = \sum x \Pr(X = x) = 2.0$$
$$\mathrm{Var}(X) = E(X^2) - [E(X)]^2 = 5 - 4 = 1$$

Practical statistics for the health sciences

Checking these values with both n and p we see that $E(X) = 2$ is simply $n \times p$, and that $Var(X) = 1$ is $n \times p(1 - p)$. It turns out that, in general, for binomial distributions

$$E(X) = n.p \quad \text{and} \quad Var(X) = n.p(1 - p)$$

These formulae are considerably easier and quicker to use than the methods described for probability distributions in general.

5.4 The Poisson distribution

Often the *rate* of occurrence of a random variable is of particular interest. For example, people concerned with the control of traffic flow might be interested in the number of vehicles that pass a particular point in a given time, or a hospital administrator might be concerned about the number of visitors passing through a ward over a given period of time. These are examples of random variables where the interest lies in the number of independent, random occurrences in a given unit of time. Other examples may include such things as the number of accidents in the workplace, the number of typing errors per page in a document, the number of flaws in a sheet of glass, and so on. These are all examples of random variables that can be modelled by the Poisson distribution. In each case the focus is on the number of occurrences of some phenomenon per unit of time, distance, area or volume.

The Poisson distribution is a discrete distribution, like the binomial, and applies whenever the occurrences, or events, occur randomly and independently of each other. It is defined by the following probability function:

$$\Pr(X = x) = \frac{e^{-\lambda}\lambda^x}{x!} \quad \text{for } x = 0, 1, 2,...$$

The expected number of occurrences or events in a given unit of time, distance, area or volume is represented by the parameter λ; if the number is not given, it can be found by multiplying the rate of the process by the given interval of time or space. For example, calls by patients to the sister station may have a rate of 20 calls per hour in a particular ward. If we are interested in the number of calls that might come in the next 15 minutes, λ is calculated as follows:

$$\lambda = 20 \times \tfrac{15}{60} = 5$$

That is, given that 20 calls would normally come in one hour, in any 15-minute period we would expect five patients to call.

The expected value and the variance of a random variable with a Poisson distribution are defined as

$$E(X) = \lambda \text{ and } Var(X) = \lambda$$

The interesting thing here is that the mean and the variance are the same.

Poisson probabilities can be determined from the probability function, or they can be found either from a set of Poisson tables or from Minitab. The Minitab printout below shows the probability distribution of a Poisson random variable with $\lambda = 2$. Use was again made of the **pdf** command used with the binomial distribution.

```
MTB > pdf;
SUBC> poisson 2.
  POISSON WITH MEAN =  2.000
   K      P( X = K)
   0       0.1353
   1       0.2707
   2       0.2707
   3       0.1804
   4       0.0902
   5       0.0361
   6       0.0120
   7       0.0034
   8       0.0009
   9       0.0002
  10       0.0000
```

Figure 5.2 Minitab printout of Poisson distribution, $\lambda = 2.0$.

```
MTB > random 250 c1;
SUBC> Poisson 1.
MTB > random 250 c2;
SUBC> Poisson 3.
MTB > random 250 c3;
SUBC> Poisson 8.
MTB > dotplot c1-c3;
SUBC> same.
Each dot represents 7 points
    :   .
    :   :
    :   :
    :   :   .                    λ = 1
    :   :   :
    :   :   :
    :   :   :   :   .
    +---------+---------+---------+---------+---------+----C1
Each dot represents 3 points
            .
        .   :       .
        :   :   .   :
        :   :   :   : .
        :   :   :   :
        :   :   :   :              λ = 3
        :   :   :   :   :
    :   :   :   :   :   :   .
    :   :   :   :   :   :   :   :   .
    +---------+---------+---------+---------+---------+----C2
Each dot represents 3 points
                    :
                    :   :
                .   :   :   :
                :   :   :   :      λ = 8
                :   :   :   :
            :   :   :   :   : . .
        :   :   :   :   :   :   :   :   :   : .
    .   .   :   :   :   :   :   :   : :   :   . .   .      .
    +---------+---------+---------+---------+---------+----C3
   0.0       3.5       7.0      10.5      14.0      17.5
```

Figure 5.3 Shapes of Poisson distributions from Minitab.

Practical statistics for the health sciences

From the printout in Figure 5.2 we see that, for $\lambda = 2$, $\Pr(X = 5) = 0.0361$. We can also see that for values of X greater than 10 the probabilities are zero (to four decimal places). To calculate the probability that $X = 10$, the formula could be used:

$$\Pr(X = 10) = \frac{e^{-2} 2^{10}}{10!} = \frac{0.1353 \times 1024}{362880} = 0.0000382$$

To four decimal places, this probability is equal to zero, as indicated on the printout.

We can obtain the shape of a Poisson distribution in the same way we did with the binomial distribution, by plotting the probability values on the vertical axis and the X values on the horizontal axis. We will use Minitab to simulate samples taken from three Poisson distributions (with $\lambda = 1$, 3, and 8) rather than draw histograms of the theoretical distributions. Figure 5.3 shows how values of λ affect the shape of the Poisson distribution. As λ increases, the Poisson distribution becomes more and more symmetrical.

Poisson probabilities occur in a great many practical situations, particularly when any form of queuing is involved, such as patients in a waiting room, accidents arriving in casualty, telephone calls to poisons information, lines at supermarket checkouts, banks and post offices, and so forth. For situations that require planning in terms of numbers of staff and their duties, an understanding of *likely* and *unlikely* scenarios is important.

EXAMPLE 5.7

The Accident and Emergency ward of the local hospital expects to treat, on average, 60 patients between 10.30 pm and 12.00 am on any Saturday night. What is the probability that more than 10 patients will arrive during a 12-minute period between 10.30 pm and 12.00 am. next Saturday night?

Solution

First obtain a value for λ. In this case $\lambda = 60 \times \frac{12}{90} = 8$. To help with this problem, a table of Poisson probabilities was obtained from Minitab using the value $\lambda = 8$.

```
MTB > pdf;
SUBC> Poisson 8.
    POISSON WITH MEAN =   8.000
```

K	P(X = K)	K	P(X = K)
0	0.0003	11	0.0722
1	0.0027	12	0.0481
2	0.0107	13	0.0296
3	0.0286	14	0.0169
4	0.0573	15	0.0090
5	0.0916	16	0.0045
6	0.1221	17	0.0021
7	0.1396	18	0.0009
8	0.1396	19	0.0004
9	0.1241	20	0.0002
10	0.0993	21	0.0001
		22	0.0000

From this table we see that $\Pr(X > 10) = 0.0722 + 0.0481 + 0.0296 + \ldots = 0.1840$

Approximating the binomial distribution

An important use for the Poisson distribution is in approximating the binomial distribution when p is small (usually < 0.05) and n is large (usually > 20). The parameter λ is then given by the mean of the binomial ie $\lambda = np$.

EXAMPLE 5.8

A sample of 30 people is randomly selected from a population in which 1% suffer from schizophrenia. Find the probability that more than two people from the sample will suffer from schizophrenia using (a) the binomial model, and (b) the Poisson model as an approximation to the binomial.

Solution

(a) From Minitab the following probability table is obtained for a binomial model with $n = 30$ and $p = 0.01$:

```
MTB > pdf;
SUBC> binomial 30 0.01.
  BINOMIAL WITH N = 30 P = 0.010000
   K      P( X = K)
   0      0.7397
   1      0.2242
   2      0.0328
   3      0.0031
   4      0.0002
   5      0.0000
```

From this table we see that $\Pr(X > 2) = 0.0031 + 0.0002 = 0.0033$. So there is only a 0.33% chance (33 chances in 10 000) that more than two people from the sample of 30 will suffer from schizophrenia.

(b) To approximate a binomial by a Poisson we use $\lambda = np$. In this case $\lambda = 0.3$. The following table is obtained from Minitab:

```
MTB > pdf;
SUBC> Poisson 0.3.
  POISSON WITH MEAN =  0.300
   K      P( X = K)
   0      0.7408
   1      0.2222
   2      0.0333
   3      0.0033
   4      0.0003
   5      0.0000
```

From this table we see that $\Pr(X > 2) = 0.0033 + 0.0003 = 0.0036$. So there is only a 0.36% chance (36 chances in 10 000) that two or more from the sample of 30 will suffer from schizophrenia.

The similarity between the results is obvious. The Poisson approximation to the binomial has resulted in a very slight overestimate of the individual probabilities in each case. The approximation would improve for larger n or smaller p-values.

Practical statistics for the health sciences

1   The probability distribution of X, the number of imperfections per 10 metres of a continuous roll of bandage of uniform width, is given as follows:

x	0	1	2	3	4
$p(x)$	0.41	0.37	0.16	0.05	0.01

Find the average number of imperfections per 10 metres of bandage.

2   The correct diagnosis of a particular illness is three times as likely to occur as an incorrect diagnosis. Find the expected number of incorrect diagnoses for the next six patients.

3   A part-time bar attendant at a local hotel supplements his wages with tips received from the customers. Usually, the more customers he serves the more in tips he is likely to make. Suppose the probabilities are $\frac{1}{12}, \frac{1}{12}, \frac{1}{4}, \frac{1}{4}, \frac{1}{6}$ and $\frac{1}{6}$ respectively that he receives $7, $9, $11, $13, $15 or $17 between 8.00 pm and 12.00 am on any Friday night. Find his expected earnings for this particular time.

4   By investing in a particular stock, there is a 30% chance of making a profit in one year of $4000, but a 70% chance of losing $1000. What is the expected gain?

5   A hospital is interested in purchasing an expensive piece of diagnostic equipment, for which the probabilities are 0.22, 0.36, 0.28 and 0.14 respectively that it will return a profit of $250 000, $150 000, break even, or incur a loss of $150 000. What is the expected profit?

6   In a gambling game a woman is paid $3 if she draws a jack or a queen and $5 if she draws a king or an ace from an ordinary deck of 52 playing cards. If she draws any other card she loses. How much should she pay to play if the game is fair (ie $E(x) = 0$)?

7   A bowl contains five tags that cannot be distinguished from one another. Three of the tags are marked $2 and the remaining two are marked $4. A player draws two tags at random from the bowl without replacement and is paid an amount equal to the sum of the values on the two tags drawn. Is this a fair game if it costs $5.60 to play?

8   The random variable X represents the number of patients in casualty, and has the following probability distribution:

x	2	3	4	5	6
$p(x)$	0.01	0.25	0.4	0.3	0.04

Find the variance of X.

9   Suppose that the probabilities are 0.4, 0.3, 0.2, and 0.1 respectively, that 0, 1, 2 or 3 power failures will hit a certain ward in a hospital in any given year. Find the mean and variance of the random variable X representing the number of power failures.

10 Hospital administration wish to insure a piece of equipment for $50 000. The insurance company estimates that a total loss may occur with probability 0.002, a 50% loss with probability 0.01, and a 25% loss with probability 0.1. Ignoring all other partial losses, what premium should the insurance company charge each year to realise an average profit of $500?

11 Let X be a random variable with the following probability distribution:

x	−2	3	5
$f(x)$	0.3	0.2	0.5

Find the standard deviation of X.

12 Fifty-five per cent of all casualty cases at a particular hospital are the result of accidents in the home. Find the probability that among the next five casualty cases:
   (a) two result from accidents in the home,
   (b) at most three result from accidents in the home.

13 A company claims that two-thirds of a particular batch of needles will be contaminated because of a faulty sealing procedure. Find the probability that among four needles inspected by nursing staff,
   (a) all four will be contaminated,
   (b) from one to three will be contaminated.

14 It is believed that 60% of people who use antidepressants initially did so for psychological reasons. Find the probability that among the next 8 users,

(a) three began taking Valium for psychological problems,

(b) at least five began taking the drug for problems that were not psychological.

15 In testing a certain type of lightweight harness for elderly patients, it is found that 25% of the harnesses fail to complete the test without tearing. Of the next 15 harnesses tested, find the probability that
(a) from three to six tear,
(b) fewer than four tear,
(c) more than five tear.

16 A survey of university nursing students reveals that 75% approve of the return of capital punishment for some offences. If 10 nursing students are randomly selected and asked their opinion, find the probability that
(a) seven to nine will approve,
(b) at most five will approve,
(c) not fewer than eight will approve,
(d) at least three will disapprove.

17 The probability that a patient will survive a delicate heart operation is 0.9. What is the probability that exactly five of the next seven patients having this operation will survive?

18 Hospital administration reports that 75% of patients reside outside the local city area. What is the probability that
(a) fewer than four of the next nine patients will reside outside the city,
(b) two or more will reside within the city?

19 A study on people's attitudes regarding tranquillisers revealed that 70% of people believe that tranquillisers only cover up the real problem. According to this study, how many people in a random sample of 20 would you expect to be of this opinion? What is the probability of obtaining exactly this number of people?

20 It is known that 40% of people inoculated with a serum are protected from a certain disease. If five people are inoculated, find the probability that
(a) none contracts the disease,
(b) fewer than two contract the disease,
(c) two or more do not contract the disease.

21 A small rural hospital averages three births per month. What is the probability that in any given month
(a) exactly five births will occur,
(b) fewer than three births will occur,
(c) at least two births will occur?

22 Secretarial staff in the admissions area of a large city hospital on average make two errors regarding each patient's personal details. What is the probability that, for the next patient,
(a) four or more errors will be made,
(b) no errors will be made?

23 A certain area in Queensland can expect six tropical cyclones per year, on average. Find the probability that in a given year this area will experience
(a) fewer than three cyclones,
(b) anywhere from six to eight cyclones.

24 Demands for a particular operation are made on average eight times per month at the local hospital. What is the probability that in any given week there will be
(a) more than two requests for the operation,
(b) no requests for the operation?
(Assume that a month contains exactly 4 weeks.)

CHAPTER OUTLINE

6.1 The normal distribution
The importance of this continuous distribution and its applications. Characteristics and mathematical properties of the normal curve. Calculating probabilities using the normal distribution and statistical tables.

6.2 The normal approximation to the binomial distribution
Criteria which must be met for it to be appropriate to use the normal distribution as an approximation to the binomial distribution.

CHAPTER SIX

Continuous density functions

After reading this chapter you should be able to:
- recognise a distribution which may be normally distributed;
- describe the shape and properties applicable to all normal curves;
- calculate standard scores;
- sketch graphs of normal distributions and locate the mean and standard deviations from the mean;
- use statistical tables to calculate probabilities for events that are normally distributed;
- describe some of the limitations of mathematical modelling;
- list the criteria which must be met to make the normal distribution an appropriate approximation to the binomial distribution; and
- calculate the mean and standard deviation of the binomial distribution, use a correction for discontinuity, and use the normal distribution as an approximation to the binomial distribution to calculate probabilities.

In many practical situations the quantities we wish to measure are *continuous random variables* like height, weight, area, air pressure, blood pressure and time. The probability of such variables assuming an exact value is theoretically zero because of the infinite number of possible values that lie between any two points on the measurement scale being used. For example, we can define an event W as follows:

W = event that the winning time for the next Melbourne marathon is 2 hours 15 minutes

There is exactly one way that this event can happen, but the number of winning times possible is infinite. Informally, we can write

$$\Pr(W) = \frac{\text{No. of favourable outcomes}}{\text{Total no. of possible outcomes}} = \frac{\text{``1''}}{\infty} \approx \text{``0''}$$

In practice, this is not a problem because no one can measure time infinitely accurately. When we say 2 hours 15 minutes (written 2.15.00) we mean between 2.14.30 and 2.15.29, depending upon the accuracy of the stopwatch or the requirements of the situation. In some sports, for example, times are measured to the nearest one thousandth of a second, while for others this level of accuracy is not required.

What we can do, however, is to calculate the probability that a continuous random variable will lie *between* any two points on the measurement scale. For example, we can calculate the probability that the finishing time for the marathon at the Sydney Olympics will lie between 2.2 and 2.3 hours. In fact there are an infinite number of winning times between 2.2 and 2.3 hours! As a consequence we conveniently represent those probabilities associated with continuous distributions by *areas under curves*. The function describing such a curve is called a probability density function (pdf); to calculate the probability of a random variable lying within a specified interval requires a technique known as *integration*. For many of the more common probability density functions, however, tables have been developed that make the task of determining these probabilities very much easier.

Figure 6.1 represents the graph of a continuous random variable X. An area under the graph has been shaded between the two values a and b. The probability that the random variable X will assume a value between the marked points is equal to the shaded area. That is, $\Pr(a \le x \le b)$ = the shaded area.

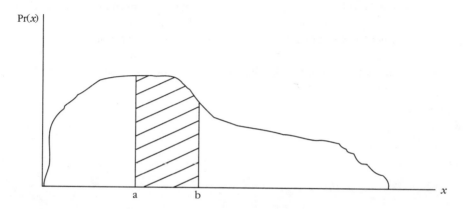

Figure 6.1 Area between two points for a continuous random variable.

Imagine letting the value *b* get closer and closer to *a*. The shaded area would therefore become smaller and smaller. At the point where *b* = *a* there would be no shaded area at all; that is, the area under the curve at the point *x* = *a* would be zero. Hence $\Pr(x = a) = 0$.

We have seen that for discrete probability distributions the sum of the probabilities is equal to 1.00. The same is true for continuous probability distributions, so the total area under the curve is equal to 1.00. The area between points *a* and *b* can thus be expressed as a proportion of the total area, and therefore can be interpreted as a probability.

It should be emphasised at this point that we are applying theoretical models to practical, physical situations, which rarely exactly fit the models being used. The advantage of using theoretical models is that they provide a mathematical framework that we can use to better understand the complexities of whatever it is that we are investigating. Also, there are many instances where the same model can be applied to different situations. This was true also for the discrete distributions encountered in the previous chapter.

There are many known continuous distributions that form an integral part of our daily lives. The accumulation of money in an account with compound interest is an example of a continuous random variable. Distributions of heights and weights are also examples of continuous random variables.

6.1   *The normal distribution*

When large numbers of measurements of people's heights are collected and arranged into a frequency distribution, a graph of the data might well look like Figure 6.2. Histograms like the one in Figure 6.2 below are often described as having a symmetrical bell-shaped distribution that is centred on the mean of the distribution.

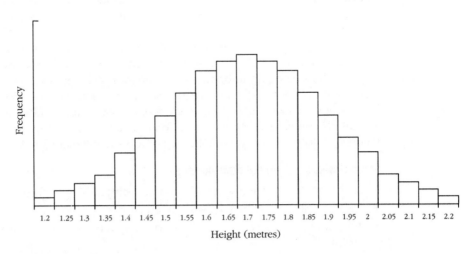

Figure 6.2 Histogram of adult heights.

If more people are included, the interval sizes become narrower and the histogram would eventually become the smooth bell-shaped curve known as the normal curve (Figure 6.3).

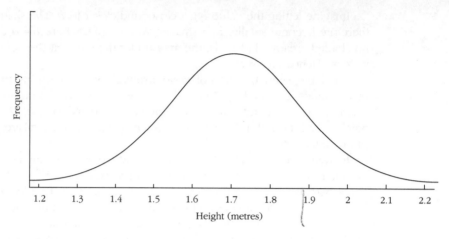

Figure 6.3 Normal curve corresponding to adult heights.

The mathematical formula that produces a bell-shaped line graph like that shown above is

$$Y = \frac{N}{\sigma\sqrt{2\pi}}\, e^{-(x-\mu)^2/2\sigma^2}$$

The value x represents any score in the distribution, and Y represents the frequency of the given value x. Notice that the value of Y depends basically upon the size (N), the centre (μ), and the spread (σ) of the distribution of scores. The constants π and e are defined as usual ($\pi = 3.1416$, and $e = 2.7183$).

Many naturally occurring variables have distributions that closely resemble the smooth, bell-shaped normal curve. Physical measurements on variables such as people's heights and weights, rainfall, manufactured parts and examination scores can often be approximated by the normal distribution. Doctors and other health professionals use properties of normal distributions to classify patients as healthy or otherwise. A healthy baby, for example, will weigh between 2750 and 3650 grams when born, and an adult should have a cholesterol level of less than 5.5 mmol/L. Readings outside these so called *normal limits* may give rise for concern.

As well as being an important distribution in the physical world, the normal distribution is the most important probability distribution in statistics, primarily because it describes the way in which *sample means* tend to be distributed. The normal distribution may also be used to accurately estimate probabilities for other theoretical distributions, given that the appropriate conditions hold.

Characteristics of normal distributions

Normal distributions have several common distinguishing features:

- they are often described as bell-shaped curves;
- they are continuous, unimodal curves, symmetric about the mean of the distribution;
- the curve is asymptotic to the horizontal axis (ie never actually touches the axis);
- theoretically, values range from $-\infty$ to $+\infty$, but in reality values of X that lie further than three standard deviations from the mean are very rare; for example, only 26 scores in 10 000 can be expected to lie further than three standard deviations from the mean; and

- there is a unique normal curve for each particular combination of a mean and a standard deviation.

The position of each curve on the horizontal axis is determined by the mean of the distribution. The shape of the curve is determined by the standard deviation (Figure 6.4).

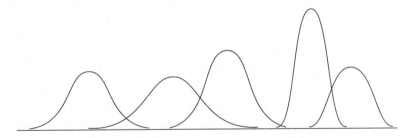

Figure 6.4 Typical normal curves with various μ and σ.

Despite the endless variety of normal curves, the basic shape remains the same. The points at which the curve changes from being concave to convex lie exactly one standard deviation either side of the mean. These points are called the *points of inflection* of the curve. If you trace over the curve with a pencil you will feel the direction of the curve change at the point of inflection.

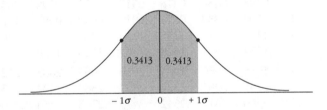

Figure 6.5 Points of inflection for the normal curve.

If we call the total area under a normal curve 1, then the proportion of the area under the curve between any two points is equal to the probability that a normally distributed variable will assume a value between those two points (Figure 6.6).

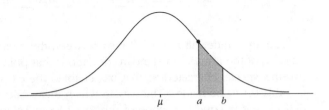

Figure 6.6 The shaded area is the probability $\Pr(a \leqslant x \leqslant b)$.

Calculating normal probabilities

Tables of values have been produced for a particular normal distribution called the standard normal distribution. This particular normal distribution has a mean of 0 and a standard deviation of 1. Data values from any normal distribution may be transformed into standardised values called *z-scores* by subtracting the mean from each *x-value* and dividing the result by the standard deviation. The distribution of the resulting z-scores has a mean of 0 and a standard deviation of 1.00, and is referred to as the standard normal distribution.

The table that has been produced for the standard normal distribution gives the areas, or probabilities, that a particular score x lies in the area between its corresponding z-score and the mean. A portion of the table is shown in Table 6.1. To use the table, a score is transformed into a z-score using the formula $z = \dfrac{x - \mu}{\sigma}$ or, as is often the case with samples, $z = \dfrac{x - \bar{x}}{s}$.

To find the probability of a value lying between $z = 0$ and $z = 1.25$ we need to locate $z = 1.25$ and read off the corresponding area, which is 0.3944. Owing to the symmetry of the distribution, the areas to the left and to the right of the mean are both 0.5, or 50% of the total area. So the area $\geq z = 1.25$ is equal to $0.50 - 0.3944 = 0.1056$. The total area $\leq z = 1.25$ is therefore equal to $0.50 + 0.3944 = 0.8944$.

Table 6.1 Portion of standard normal probability tables.

Areas under the standard normal probability distribution

z	.00	.01	.02	.03	.04	.05	.06	.07	.08	.09
.0	.0000	.0040	.0080	.0120	.0160	.0199	.0239	.0279	.0319	.0359
.1	.0398	.0438	.0478	.0517	.0557	.0596	.0636	.0675	.0714	.0753
.2	.0793	.0832	.0871	.0910	.0948	.0987	.1026	.1064	.1103	.1141
.3	.1179	.1217	.1255	.1293	.1331	.1368	.1406	.1443	.1480	.1517
.4	.1554	.1591	.1628	.1664	.1700	.1736	.1772	.1808	.1844	.1879
.5	.1915	.1950	.1985	.2019	.2054	.2088	.2123	.2157	.2190	.2224
.6	.2257	.2291	.2324	.2357	.2389	.2422	.2454	.2486	.2518	.2549
.7	.2580	.2611	.2642	.2673	.2703	.2734	.2764	.2794	.2823	.2852
.8	.2881	.2910	.2939	.2967	.2995	.3023	.3051	.3078	.3106	.3133
.9	.3159	.3186	.3212	.3238	.3264	.3289	.3315	.3340	.3365	.3389
1.0	.3413	.3438	.3461	.3485	.3508	.3531	.3554	.3577	.3599	.3621
1.1	.3643	.3665	.3686	.3708	.3729	.3749	.3770	.3790	.3810	.3830
1.2	.3849	.3869	.3888	.3907	.3925	.3944	.3962	.3980	.3997	.4015
1.3	.4032	.4049	.4066	.4082	.4099	.4115	.4131	.4147	.4162	.4177
1.4	.4192	.4207	.4222	.4236	.4251	.4265	.4279	.4292	.4306	.4319

The area under all normal curves between the mean and any other point is a function of the number of standard deviations that point lies away from the mean. It is this special characteristic that has enabled the calculation of the probabilities in Table 6.1 to be made. (The way in which these calculations have been made is difficult and beyond the scope of this text.) From Table 6.1 it can be verified that the following approximations hold for all normal distributions:

- 68% of the distribution lies within one standard deviation of the mean,
- 95% of the distribution lies within two standard deviations of the mean, and
- 99.7% of the distribution lies within three standard deviations of the mean.

Practical statistics for the health sciences

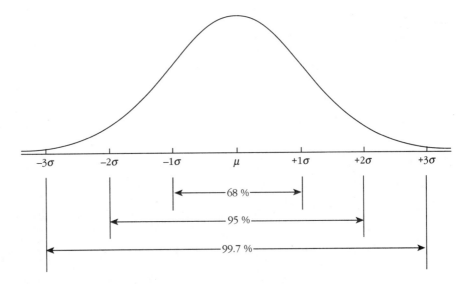

Figure 6.7 Areas under a normal curve.

Modelling normality

While we use the normal distribution to represent physical measurements that have been grouped into a frequency distribution, no set of real-life data can be expected to conform exactly to this distribution. Real data does not vary between $-\infty$ and $+\infty$, and limitations of measuring instruments effectively eliminate many other potential values. It is impossible, for example, for birth weights to be negative, and similarly for many other physical measurements. Even so, the normal distribution still provides us with good approximations to real-life data.

So when we say that a random variable is normally distributed, we mean that a frequency distribution of its possible outcomes can be approximated quite well using a normal probability distribution. Hence the normal curve is a model.

EXAMPLE   6.1

Pulse rates are approximately normally distributed with $\mu = 72$ and $\sigma = 5$. Use the normal tables to find the following probabilities that a person chosen at random will have a pulse rate:
(a) greater than 75; (b) greater than 65; (c) between 65 and 80.

Solution
(a) The diagram (right) shows the required area.
We have $x = 75$, $\mu = 72$, and $\sigma = 5$.

Therefore $z = \dfrac{75 - 72}{5} = \dfrac{3}{5} = 0.6$

From the tables $\Pr(0 \le z \le 0.6) = 0.2257$
Therefore $\Pr(x > 75) = 0.5 - 0.2257 = 0.2743$

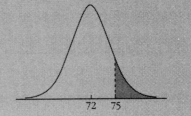

EXAMPLE 6.1   cont.

(b) The diagram (right) shows the required area
We have $x = 65$, $\mu = 72$, and $\sigma = 5$.

Therefore $z = \dfrac{65 - 72}{5} = -\dfrac{7}{5} = -1.4$

From the tables $\Pr(-1.4 \leq z \leq 0) = 0.4192$
Therefore $\Pr(x > 65) = 0.5 + 0.4192 = 0.9192$

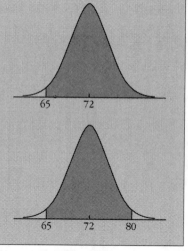

(c) From (b) $\Pr(65 < x < 72) = 0.4192$

For $x = 80$, we have $z = \dfrac{80 - 72}{5} = \dfrac{8}{5} = 1.6$

From the tables $\Pr(0 \leq z \leq 1.6) = 0.4452$
Therefore $\Pr(65 < x < 80) = 0.4192 + 0.4452 = 0.8644$

6.2 The normal approximation to the binomial distribution

Many real-life situations are aptly described by the binomial distribution, but the binomial tables rarely extend beyond $n = 20$ and calculations are tedious. Fortunately, in many instances the normal distribution can be used to obtain fairly good approximations to binomial probabilities. The normal approximation works best when the probability of success is close to 0.50, and the approximation improves as n gets larger. For large values of n (ie $n > 200$) the need for p-values close to 0.5 diminishes. One generally accepted rule of thumb is that both np and $n(1 - p)$ should be greater than or equal to 5 in order to use the normal approximation.

Since the binomial distribution is discrete and the normal distribution is continuous, we need to use a *continuity correction factor* as a form of adjustment. For example, continuous values in the range 12.5 to 13.5 would relate to the discrete, or integer, value of 13. So to find the binomial probability of exactly 13 successes from 20 trials, we could use a normal approximation based on the probability of obtaining a value between 12.5 and 13.5 successes. To find the probability of between 13 and 15 successes inclusive we would need to use the interval 12.5 to 15.5. The histogram for the binomial distribution with $n = 20$ and $p = 0.5$ is shown in Figure 6.8 with the corresponding normal distribution having mean $\mu = np = 10$ and variance $\sigma^2 = np(1 - p) = 5$. (See mean and variance for a binomial distribution in Section 5.2.)

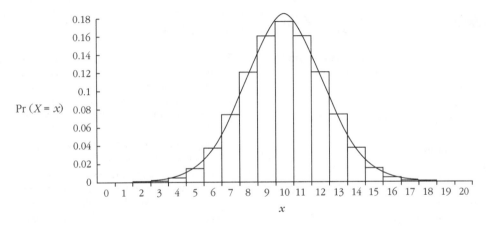

Figure 6.8 Normal approximation of binomial.

EXAMPLE **6.2**

Police records show that, on an average Saturday night, 1 in every 10 drivers will have a blood alcohol content above the legal limit. If 500 drivers are to be randomly tested next Saturday night, what is the probability that the number of drivers exceeding the legal limit will be (a) less than 40; and (b) more than 50, but less than 60.

Solution

Using the normal approximation we have
$\mu = np = 500 \times 0.1 = 50$, and $\sigma = \sqrt{np(1 - p)} = \sqrt{500 \times 0.1 \times 0.9} = 6.708$

(a) For $x < 40$ we require $\Pr(x \leq 39.5)$. $z = \dfrac{39.5 \ 1 \ 50}{6.708} = -1.565$

From the tables, $\Pr(-1.57 \leq z \leq 0) = 0.4418$
Therefore $\Pr(x < 40) = 0.5 - 0.4418 = 0.0582$

(b) For x more than 50 and less than 60, we require $\Pr(50.5 \leq x \leq 59.5)$

For $x = 50.5$, $z = \dfrac{50.5 - 50}{6.708} = 0.07$, and tabled area $= 0.0279$

For $x = 59.5$, $z = \dfrac{59.5 - 50}{6.708} = 1.42$, and tabled area $= 0.4222$

Therefore $\Pr(50.5 \leq x \leq 59.5) = 0.0279 + 0.4222 = 0.4501$

1 Given a standard normal distribution, find the area under the curve which lies
  (a) to the left of $z = 1.43$,
  (b) to the right of $z = -0.89$,
  (c) between $z = -2.16$ and $z = -0.65$,
  (d) to the left of $z = -1.39$,
  (e) greater than $z = 1.96$,
  (f) between $z = -0.48$ and $z = 1.74$.

2 Find the value of z if the area under a standard normal curve
  (a) greater than z is 0.3632,
  (b) less than z is 0.1131,
  (c) between 0 and z with $z > 0$ is 0.4838,
  (d) between $-z$ and z, with $z > 0$ is 0.95.

3 We know that a set of data fits a standard normal distribution. In each case below find the value of k that divides the distribution so that
  (a) $\Pr(z < k) = 0.0427$,
  (b) $\Pr(z > k) = 0.2946$,
  (c) $\Pr(-0.93 < z < k) = 0.7235$.

4 Given a normal distribution with $\mu = 30$ and $\sigma = 6$, find
  (a) the proportion greater than $x = 17$,
  (b) the area to the left of $x = 22$,
  (c) the percentage of the distribution between $x = 32$ and 41.

5 Certain strips of gauze bandage have an average length of 30 cm with a standard deviation of 2 cm. Assuming that the lengths of gauze are normally distributed, what percentage are
  (a) longer than 31.7 cm,
  (b) between 29.3 and 33.5 cm in length,
  (c) shorter than 25.5 cm.

6 A coffee machine in the hospital cafeteria is regulated so that it delivers 200 mL per cup on average. If the amount delivered is normally distributed with a standard deviation of 15 mL,
  (a) what fraction of the cups will contain more than 224 mL?
  (b) what is the probability of a cup containing between 191 and 209 mL?
  (c) how many cups will overflow if 230 mL cups are used for the next 1000 drinks?
  (d) below what value do we get the smallest 25% of the drinks?

7 A student nurse drives daily from where she lives in the city to the hospital where she works. On average the one-way trip takes 24 minutes with a standard deviation of 3.8 minutes. Assume that the distribution of one-way travel times is normal.
  (a) What is the probability that a trip will take at least half an hour?
  (b) If she is supposed to start at 9.00 am and she leaves home at 8.45 am, what percentage of the time will she be late for work?
  (c) If she leaves home at 8.35 am and coffee is served at the hospital from 8.50 until 9.00 am, what is the probability she will miss coffee?
  (d) At what time should she leave home if she does not want to be late more than 5% of the time?

8 If a set of nursing examination results are normally distributed with a mean of 74 and a standard deviation of 7.9, find
  (a) the lowest possible pass mark if 10% of the students are failed,
  (b) the highest possible B if only 5% of students are given an A,
  (c) the lowest possible B if 10% of the students are given As and the next 25% are given Bs.

9 In a statistics examination the average mark was 82 and the standard deviation was 5. All students with marks from 88 to 94 received a B grade. If the grades are normally distributed and eight students received a B grade, how many students sat the examination?

10 The heights of 500 male nursing students are normally distributed with a mean of 174.5 cm and a standard deviation of 6.9 cm. If the heights are recorded to the nearest half centimetre, how many of these students would you expect to have heights
  (a) less than 160 cm,
  (b) from 171.5 to 182 cm inclusive,
  (c) equal to 175 cm,
  (d) greater than or equal to 188 cm?

11 Weights of new-born babies are normally distributed with a mean of 3300 g and a standard deviation of 400 g. If measurements are recorded to the nearest gram find the percentage of new-born babies with weights

(a) over 4000 g,

(b) at most 3950 g,

(c) from 2500 to 4100 g inclusive,

(d) that differ by more than 1.5 σ from μ,

(e) that differ by less than 0.75 σ from μ?

12 The entrance examination results of 600 students seeking places in nursing courses were normally distributed with $\mu = 105$ and $\sigma = 12$. If a requirement of the nursing course administrators is a score of at least 95, how many of these students will be rejected?

13 The average life of a major piece of hospital equipment is considered to be 10 years with a standard deviation of 2 years, and is assumed to be normally distributed. If the equipment fails while still under guarantee it will be replaced free of charge. If the manufacturer is willing to replace the equipment in only 3% of cases, how long should the guarantee period be?

14 Evaluate Pr$(1 \leq x \leq 4)$ for a binomial variable with $n = 15$ and $p = 0.2$ using

(a) the binomial tables,

(b) a normal approximation method.

Hint: Remember the correction for discontinuity.

15 A particular massage technique is 50% successful in relieving stress in patients. For 400 patients, use the normal approximation to the binomial to find the probability of relieving stress

(a) for between 185 and 210 patients,

(b) for exactly 205 patients,

(c) for less than 176 or more than 227.

16 A pair of dice is rolled 180 times. What is the probability that a total of 7 occurs

(a) at least 25 times,

(b) between 33 and 41 times inclusive,

(c) exactly 30 times?

17 The probability that a patient recovers from a delicate heart operation is 0.9. Of the next 100 patients having this operation what is the probability that

(a) the success rate is 95% or more,

(b) the success rate is less than 85%?

18 If 75% of people believe that tranquillisers do have a calming effect, then of the next 80 people interviewed, what is the probability that

(a) at least 50 are of this opinion,

(b) at most 56 are of this opinion,

(c) no more than 20 disagree?

19 A drug company claims that a new drug used to treat a certain blood disorder is successful, on average, 80% of the time. To check this, use of the drug was monitored for a sample of 100 patients and it was decided to accept the claim if 75 or more of the patients were cured.

(a) What is the probability that the claim will be rejected when the cure rate is in fact 80%?

(b) What is the probability that the claim will be accepted if the cure rate is really only 70%?

20 It is believed that, on an average weekend night in a particular area, 1 out of every 10 drivers on the road is drunk. If 400 drivers are randomly checked next Saturday night, what is the probability that the number of drunk drivers will be

(a) less than 32?

(b) more than 49?

(c) at least 35 but less than 47?

Progress review 2

1   Our alphabet contains 26 letters, consisting of the 5 vowels and 21 consonants. Let the two events *A* and *B* below be defined as follows:
    A = the event that a randomly selected letter is a vowel
    B = the event that a randomly selected letter lies between the letters *a* and *m* inclusive.
    (a) Calculate the following probabilities:
       (i) Pr(*A*)   (ii) Pr(*B*)   (iii) Pr(*A* and *B*)
       (iv) Pr(*A*|*B*)   (v) Pr(*A* or *B*)
    (b) Show that Pr (*A* and *B*) = Pr(*A*) Pr(*B*|*A*).

2   A survey of 200 nursing students found that
    • 50 students had worked in a children's ward,
    • 20 students had worked in both a children's ward and an emergency ward, and
    • 50 students had not worked in either.
    (a) Summarise the information in the form of a Venn diagram.
    (b) Use the diagram to find the probability that a randomly selected student will:
       (i) have only worked in a children's ward,
       (ii) not have worked in an emergency ward,
       (iii) have worked in either a children's ward or an emergency ward,
       (iv) have worked in a children's ward given previous experience in an emergency ward.
    (c) Given that a randomly selected student had not worked in a children's ward, what is the probability that the same student had not worked in an emergency ward also?

3   A study was undertaken of the performances of mathematics students in recent university examinations and how their results related to the mathematics studied in Year 12. The results are summarised in the table below. Assume that no student studied more than one of the three areas listed.

University result	Year 12 maths studied		
	General	Statistics	Calculus
Pass	10	40	35
Fail	40	20	5

    (a) What proportion of students studied Statistics?
    (b) What proportion of students failed their university examination?
    (c) What proportion of the Calculus students failed their university examination?
    (d) Given that a randomly selected student failed their university examination, what is the probability of that student having studied Statistics at Year 12?

4   Let the random variable *X* represent the number of times that power fluctuations or failures affect the operation of sensitive monitoring equipment in an intensive care ward of a particular hospital in any given week. Let *X* have the following probability distribution:

X	0	1	2	3	4
Pr(*X* = *x*)	0.70	0.20	0.07	0.02	0.01

    (a) What is the probability of there being:
       (i) two or more power failures in any given week,
       (ii) more than four failures in any given week?
    (b) Find the expected number of power failures in any given week.

Practical statistics for the health sciences

(c) Calculate the standard deviation for the distribution.

(d) How many power failures can be expected in any given year?

5   A survey of student nurses revealed that 40% smoked cigarettes regularly. If 10 students are chosen at random, find the probability that:

(a) from seven to nine inclusive regularly smoke cigarettes,

(b) no more than five regularly smoke cigarettes,

(c) at least five do not regularly smoke cigarettes,

(d) none smoke cigarettes regularly.

6   (a) Given a normal distribution with $\mu = 20$ and $\sigma = 4$, find

   (i)   the normal curve area to the right of $x = 17$,

   (ii) the normal curve area between $x = 17$ and 24,

   (iii) the value of z if the area to the left of z is 0.7500,

   (iv) the x-value above which only 5% of the distribution lies.

(b) The average number of matches in a box of matches is 50. Assume that the distribution of the actual number of matches per box is approximately normal, with a standard deviation of 1.5 matches. (Hint: as the number of matches in a box is discrete, you should use the continuity correction factor.)

   (i)   What proportion of match boxes will contain less than 48 matches?

   (ii) From a sample of 100 boxes of matches, how many boxes would you expect to contain from 51 to 54 matches?

   (iii) What is the probability of a box containing 54 or more matches?

   (iv) What should the standard deviation be reduced to if no more than 5% of the match boxes produced are to contain less than 48 matches?

CHAPTER SEVEN

Correlation

LEARNING OBJECTIVES

After reading this chapter you should be able to:

- correctly plot a scatter diagram for two variables;
- use Minitab or formulae to calculate linear correlation coefficients; and
- interpret linear correlations in the context of the problem set.

In our day-to-day lives we often gain the impression, based upon our informal observations, that two variables may be related in some way. For example, it was observed that patients suffering from lung diseases were often also smokers. Studies were carried out by many researchers to see if this was a chance observation, or whether in fact there was a significant, predictable relationship between the number of cigarettes smoked and the occurrence of different types of lung diseases. Similar investigations include:

- the depletion of the ozone layer of the atmosphere and the increasing incidence of skin cancers,
- underground nuclear explosions and the perceived increased frequency of earthquakes, and
- the use of food additives and the occurrence of bowel cancers.

In this chapter we investigate some of the statistical methods that enable us to measure the relationship between two variables. *Correlation* and *regression* are procedures describing the relationship between a set of paired scores representing variables such as aptitude and examination results, blood alcohol content and reaction time, the rankings of two independent judges at a wine show, and weights of mothers and their newborn babies. The major purpose of collecting bivariate data (data dealing with two variables) is to consider questions such as:

- Are the variables related?
- What form of relationship is indicated by the data?
- Can we quantify the strength of their relationship?
- Can we predict one variable from the other?

7.1 Scatterplots

A scatterplot is a graph that plots the paired measurements of one variable against another. These graphs are very easy and quick to construct, and are particularly useful in determining the nature of the relationship between the two variables. Figure 7.1 shows two points that have been plotted on a pair of axes, with mother's weight in kilograms on the horizontal axis, and infant's weight in grams on the vertical axis. One mother weighed 60 kg and had a 3750 g infant, while the other mother weighed 72 kg and had an infant weighing 4000 g.

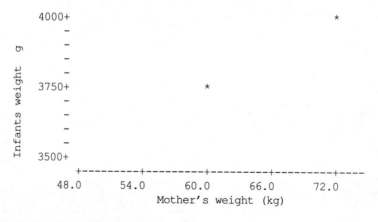

Figure 7.1 An example of a simple scatterplot.

When many of these points are plotted, a *pattern* may begin to emerge, and it is the nature of this pattern that is of interest. Usually, the stronger the relationship between the two variables, the more evident the pattern will be.

EXAMPLE **7.1**

The following results were achieved by 16 students undertaking both theoretical and clinical examinations as part of a university nursing course. Construct a scatterplot of the data and comment upon its shape.

| Theory % | 75 | 30 | 73 | 40 | 94 | 85 | 95 | 79 | 64 | 87 | 70 | 60 | 75 | 73 | 90 | 74 |
| Clinical % | 58 | 25 | 67 | 35 | 89 | 73 | 90 | 67 | 58 | 83 | 70 | 50 | 67 | 74 | 68 | 60 |

Solution

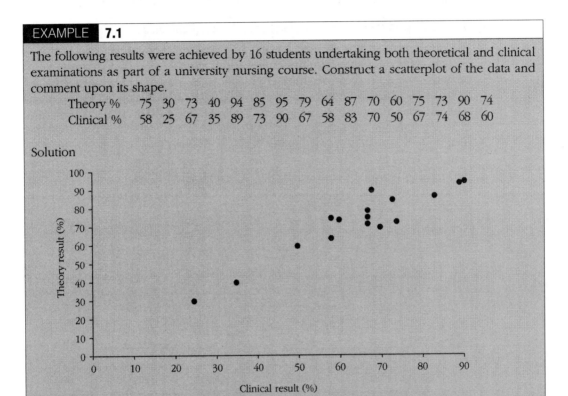

The scatterplot shows that the points seem to lie along a straight line extending from the bottom left corner to the top right corner. We say that the direction of the relationship is *positive*, and the nature of the relationship is appears to be *linear*.

7.2   Correlation

Correlation coefficients quantify the *strength* and *direction* of a relationship that may exist between two variables. At this stage we will restrict ourselves to *linear* relationships. Correlation coefficients are expressed as numbers from −1.0 to +1.0. Negative correlation coefficients indicate negative relationships, where values of one variable tend to decrease as the values of the second variable increase. For example, as the average temperature increases, the amount of electricity or gas used for heating decreases. Positive coefficients indicate positive relationships, where values of both variables increase (or decrease) together. For example, as temperatures increase so do sales of ice-creams. Correlation coefficients that are close to ±1.0 imply that the relationship between the two variables is a very strong one. If the correlation coefficient is close to zero then the linear relationship between the variables is very weak.

Correlation coefficients can be used as a basis for prediction and for assessing the reliability of testing instruments. Two of the most widely used correlation coefficients are Pearson's product-moment correlation coefficient, denoted by the symbol r, and Spearman's rank correlation coefficient, denoted by the symbol r_s.

Pearson's product-moment correlation coefficient (Pearson's r)

For linear relationships the most commonly used correlation coefficient is Pearson's r. This coefficient takes positive values if the variables are directly related and negative values if they are inversely related. The possible range of values for Pearson's r is from −1.0 through to +1.0. A correlation coefficient of plus or minus one indicates that the values lie in a straight line, while a value close to ±1 indicates a strong linear relationship. On the other hand, a value close to zero indicates that there is not a linear relationship between the two variables. This may mean that the variables are not related in any way, or that there may be a *non-linear* relationship between the two variables. A scatterplot of the data will usually help interpret the correlation coefficient. Figure 7.2 shows some scatterplots for different values of r.

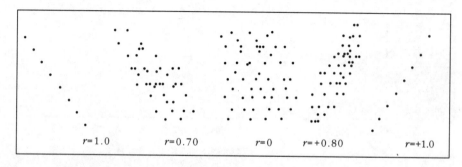

Figure 7.2 Scatterplots for various values of Pearson's r.

It is important to look at a scatterplot of the data, since a low value of Pearson's r indicates only a lack of a linear relationship between the two variables. There may be a curved relationship or some other relationship that is non-linear. In these instances a linear correlation coefficient is not suitable unless the raw scores have been *transformed* to make them linear. However, interpretations can become more complicated when dealing with transformed data. At this level we will not consider using transformations in any great detail.

Calculating Pearson's r

Correlation coefficients are best found using computer packages like Minitab. The practical and theory test scores for the 16 students used in Example 7.1 were put into columns 1 and 2 of a Minitab worksheet and a scatterplot and the correlation coefficient were obtained.

The command PLOT was used to obtain the scatterplot, with the column for the vertical axis mentioned first of all. The command CORRELATE was used to obtain a value for Pearson's r. The value of +0.940 indicates a very strong positive relationship between the theory and practical test scores for this group of students. That is, high practical scores tend to be associated with high theory scores.

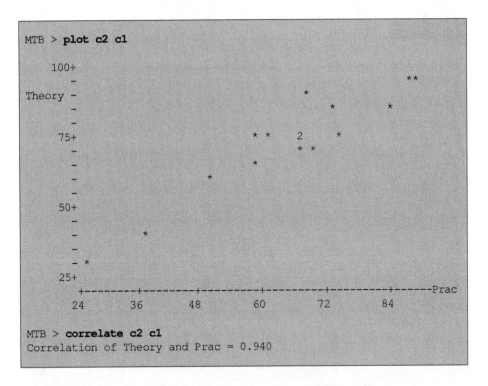

Figure 7.3 Minitab printout showing scatterplot and correlation coefficient.

The calculation of Pearson's r relies initially upon determining the following quantities from the raw data:

$$n, \Sigma x, \Sigma y, \Sigma xy, \Sigma x^2 \text{ and } \Sigma y^2$$

which are substituted into the following formula:

$$r = \frac{n\Sigma xy - \Sigma x . \Sigma y}{\sqrt{(n\Sigma x^2 - [\Sigma x]^2)(n\Sigma y^2 - [\Sigma y]^2)}}$$

Care needs to be taken with this formula, particularly with the denominator, as the square root is often forgotten in the final stages of the calculation. Example 7.2 uses the formula to calculate Pearson's correlation coefficient.

EXAMPLE	7.2

A random sample of cars, all of the same model, engine size, etc. were driven through city traffic at different speeds for a distance of 100 km. The amount of fuel used by each vehicle was recorded. The results are listed below:

Speed (km/h)	10	20	15	20	60	90	75	55	30	40
Fuel (L)	12	11	11	12	10	11	9.5	10	11	11

EXAMPLE **7.2** **cont.**

```
 12.0+    *    *
      -
Fuel  -
      -         *  *    *   *                            *
      -
 10.5+
      -
      -
      -                       *  *
      -                     *
      +----------+----------+----------+--------kph
      0         25         50         75
```

The scatterplot suggests a negative relationship exists between these variables. That is, the correlation coefficient should be negative.

Solution

$n = 10$, $\Sigma x = 415$, $\Sigma y = 108.5$, $\Sigma xy\, 4367.5$

$\Sigma x^2 = 23975$ and $\Sigma y^2 = 1183.25$

$$r = \frac{10(4367.5) - 415 \times 108.5}{\sqrt{[10(23975) - 415^2][10(1183.25) - 108.5^2]}}$$

$$r = \frac{43675 - 45027.5}{\sqrt{[239750 - 172225][11832.5 - 11772.25]}} = \frac{-1352.5}{\sqrt{67525 \times 60.25}}$$

$$r = \frac{-1352.5}{\sqrt{4068381.25}} = -0.6705$$

Spearman's rank–difference correlation coefficient

In a social science context it is common to have to deal with data which is only of ordinal scaling. For example, nurses' opinions about which aspects of their work they find stressful could produce ordinal data. Such data, which has only been *ranked*, can be dealt with by using Spearman's rank correlation coefficient, r_s, commonly referred to as *Spearman's rho*. Like Pearson's r, Spearman's r_s varies between –1.0 and +1.0, with 0 indicating the absence of a relationship.

To calculate Spearman's r_s:

1 Rank the scores for each variable separately. When there are 'ties' in the scores, average their ranks and give this average rank to each one of the tied scores.

2 Calculate the differences between the rankings for each pair of scores. These differences we denote by the letter d.

3 Square the differences and add them up (ie Σd^2).

4 Calculate Spearman's rank–difference correlation coefficient according to the formula:

$$r_s = 1 - \frac{6\Sigma d^2}{n(n^2 - 1)}$$

where n represents the number of pairs of observations.

When establishing rankings for a set of data you can do so in either ascending or descending order. When dealing with more than one variable you will need to be consistent. Example 7.3 ranks the data in ascending order; that is, it starts with the lowest value and works up to the largest value.

EXAMPLE **7.3**

Rank the following values from lowest to highest.

Raw Scores   65 60 58 72 60 70 65 70 75 80 55 70 68 63 67

Solution

Initially it helps to write the scores in ascending order.

Scores	55	58	60	60	63	65	65	67	68	70	70	70	72	75	80
Ranks	1	2	3.5	3.5	5	6.5	6.5	8	9	11	11	11	13	14	15

Notice in Example 7.3 that there were two values equal to 60, and these values have a ranking that is the average of rankings 3 and 4. Similarly with the ranking of 6.5 given to the two values equal to 65. The ranking for the three values equal to 70 was obtained by averaging the rankings 10, 11 and 12. To check the accuracy of your rankings, the following relationship should hold true:

$$\Sigma \text{rankings} = \frac{n(n+1)}{2}$$

In Example 7.3, Σrankings = $1 + 2 + 3.5 + \ldots = 120$, and $\frac{n(n+1)}{2} = \frac{15 \times 16}{2} = 120$. Therefore the allocation of rankings is correct.

Example 7.4 involves assessing student nurses by using an examination as well as a ranking by a clinical supervisor. The purpose is to see if there is any correlation between the examination scores and the rankings given by the supervisor. If a perfect positive relationship exists between the two forms of measurement, their corresponding ranks would be identical. A perfect negative relationship between the two groups of scores would imply that corresponding ranks would be opposite. That is, the highest rankings in one group would be paired with the lowest rankings in the other group. In this case, Spearman's correlation coefficient is measured on the basis of the *differences between the rankings*.

EXAMPLE **7.4**

Examination scores and clinical rankings for a sample of ten students were obtained with the following results:

Student	a	b	c	d	e	f	g	h	i	j
Exam	48	37	30	45	31	24	28	18	35	15
Ranking	10	9	4	7	9	4	3	1	8	2

What is the nature of the correlation between the examination results and the rankings provided by the clinical supervisor?

EXAMPLE **7.4**   **cont.**

Solution

(a) Separately rank the two sets of scores.

Exam.	48	37	30	45	31	24	28	18	35	15
Rank	10	8	5	9	6	3	4	2	7	1

Ability	10	9	4	7	9	4	3	1	8	2
Rank	10	8.5	4.5	6	8.5	4.5	3	1	7	2

(b) Find the differences between the pairs of rankings

Exam Rank	10	8	5	9	6	3	4	2	7	1
Ability Rank	10	8.5	4.5	6	8.5	4.5	3	1	7	2
Difference	0	−0.5	0.5	3	−2.5	−1.5	1	1	0	−1

(c) Calculate the sum of the squared differences

$$\sum d^2 = 0^2 + (-0.5)^2 + (0.5)^2 + 3^2 + \ldots = 0 + 0.25 + 0.25 + 9 + \ldots + 1 = 21$$

(d) $r_s = 1 - \dfrac{6 \times 21}{10(100 - 1)} = 1 - \dfrac{126}{990} = 0.8727$

There is a strong positive correlation between the two forms of measurement.
The same result can be obtained by entering the ranks into a calculator or Minitab and, using the appropriate keystrokes or Minitab commands, obtaining the value for r_s.

7.3   *Interpreting correlation coefficients*

Correlation coefficients measure the strength of the mathematical relationship between two variables. This may or may not correspond to a practical real-life link between the variables. A high correlation between two variables does not necessarily mean that one causes the other. For example, suppose that a school nurse noticed a positive relationship between the number of stomach upsets reported and the quantity of water drunk by students from the school taps. In fact, the cause of the stomach upsets was not the amount of water drunk, but rather the fact that the students had been eating blackberries sprayed with herbicide.

So an observed correlation between two variables simply means that variation in one is associated in some way with variation in the other; it does not necessarily mean that a cause-and-effect relationship exists. Often a third variable can be the hidden cause of an observed correlation. This is sometimes referred to as a *spurious* correlation. For example, the weight of a car and its fuel consumption probably have a high positive correlation, but to what degree does this correlation depend upon the person driving the car? The manner in which a car is driven can have a marked effect upon fuel consumption. Researchers must not jump to conclusions; high correlations do suggest avenues for further investigation, and often common sense can determine if a correlation is spurious or not.

The classification of correlation values as *high*, *medium* or *low* must be related to the context within which they occur. Consider what a correlation of 0.90 does not mean: it does not mean that the two variables are associated 90% of the time, and nor does it mean that they are associated twice as much as variables with a correlation coefficient of 0.45. Correlations are a measure of the strength of the relationship — interpretation must be practical. For example, it is very common to get coefficients of 0.90 or higher when measuring test–retest reliability. In this context a coefficient of 0.80 would be considered quite low and raise doubts as to the reliability of the particular instrument. However, in a large-scale study of heart disease, where many factors are measured, a correlation of even 0.3 may be considered sufficiently high to warrant further investigation. There can be no single scheme for interpreting correlation coefficients which will be applicable in all cases.

1 Compute and interpret the correlation coefficient for the following marks for six randomly selected third-year nursing students.

Statistics	70 92 80 74 65 83
Nursing Practice	74 84 63 87 78 90

2 The following measurements were made in a study of the relationship between the weight and chest size of infants at birth:

Weight (kg)	Chest size (cm)
2.75	29.5
2.15	26.3
4.41	32.2
5.52	36.5
3.21	27.2
4.32	27.7
2.31	28.3
3.71	28.7
4.30	30.3

(a) Calculate the correlation coefficient between these two variables.

(b) What percentage of the variation in infant chest sizes is explained by differences in weight?

3 A study was conducted to investigate the relationship between cigarette smoking and sick leave. The average number of cigarettes smoked daily and the number of days absent from work in the last year due to illness was determined for 12 nurses at a particular hospital.

Subject	Cigarettes smoked	Days absent
1	0	1
2	0	3
3	0	8
4	10	10
5	13	2
6	20	14
7	27	2
8	35	6
9	35	12
10	44	16
11	53	10
12	60	16

(a) Construct a scatterplot for the data.

(b) Calculate the value of Pearson's r.

(c) Eliminate the data from the non-smokers (ie the first three subjects) and recalculate Pearson's r for the remaining subjects. What effect has decreasing the range of the data had on r?

(d) What percentage of the variability in the number of days absent is accounted for by the number of cigarettes smoked daily? Of what use is this value?

4 A stress questionnaire relating to 15 life events was given to large samples from two cultural groups in Australia. Researchers were interested in determining whether there was cross-cultural agreement on the relative amount of adjustment each life-event entailed. The higher the points, the greater the adjustment required. After each subject had assigned points to each life-event, the points for each event were averaged. The results were as follows:

Life event	Group 1	Group 2
Death of spouse	100	80
Divorce	73	95
Marital separation	65	85
Jail term	63	52
Personal injury	53	72
Marriage	50	60
Fired from work	47	40
Retirement	45	30
Pregnancy	40	38
Sex difficulties	39	42
Business problems	39	36
Trouble with in-laws	29	41
Trouble with boss	23	35
Vacation	13	16
Christmas	12	10

(a) Assume the data are at least of interval scaling and compute the correlation between the ratings of the two cultural groups.

(b) Assume the data are only of ordinal scaling and compute the correlation between the ratings of the two cultural groups.

5 Which of the following are incorrect interpretations of a correlation coefficient, and why?

(a) The strength of the association between two test forms L and M is 0.96.

(b) The correlation between height and weight at age 6 is 0.40; this is twice as high as that at age 16, when $r = 0.20$.

(c) There is a medium correlation of 0.67 between the age at which babies can roll over and the age at which they can sit up alone.

(d) We can conclude from the high correlation between level of motivation and number of elective offices sought, that office-seeking behaviour is caused at least in part by motivation.

6 A written test was intended to measure the efficiency of nurses in an emergency situation. The test was given to a sample of 12 nurses and results from the test were compared to rankings of the same nurses given by two experienced nurses who were experts in the area. The results appear in the table below: higher scores represent greater efficiency.

Written test	Expert A	Expert B
48	12	9
37	11	12
30	4	5
45	7	8
31	10	11
24	8	7
28	3	4
18	1	1
35	9	6
15	2	2
42	6	10
22	5	3

(a) What is the correlation between the rankings of the two experts?

(b) What are the correlations between the scores from the written test and the rankings of each expert?

7 The following data represent the results of 10 students in nursing theory and practical examinations.

Theory   5 4 5 2 2 6 1 5 6 4
Practical 14 6 8 2 8 14 4 4 10 10

(a) Construct a scatterplot of the data and use it to estimate the correlation between the theory and practical marks.

(b) Calculate Spearman's and Pearson's correlation coefficients.

8 Use the following data to find the linear correlation between the two variables. Comment on what you find.

Radius of ulcer (mm)	Time of healing (weeks)
2.4	1.5
2.8	4.3
5.6	7.8
2.7	2.4
8.6	10.3
3.5	4.9
6.6	5.9
3.4	2.1
8.4	7.3
5.7	6.1

9 The following table contains data for a group of trainee nurses who were tested on nursing theory. The same students were also given a rating by their clinical supervisors in a hospital setting. Is it likely that the test could be used in place of the supervisors' comments?

Student	Rating	Test
1	Good	86
2	Fair	58
3	Very poor	50
4	Excellent	95
5	Very good	84
6	Average	63
7	Average	70
8	Fair to good	58
9	Weak	47
10	Average	60
11	Good to very good	70

10 In the following pairs of observations, x represents the intensity of a sound stimulus and y is the reaction time required by the subject before responding to the sound.

x	y	x	y
1.3	1.70	6.2	0.61
2.1	1.62	6.9	0.70
2.4	1.48	7.4	0.44
3.0	1.00	7.4	0.31
3.8	1.19	8.1	0.33
4.5	1.23	9.6	0.30
5.1	0.80	10.0	0.18
5.7	0.59	10.9	0.15
6.0	0.35		

Comment on the strength and the direction of the relationship between these two variables.

CHAPTER EIGHT

Linear regression

LEARNING OBJECTIVES

After reading this chapter you should be able to:

- decide whether a linear regression model would be appropriate for a given set of data;
- use Minitab or formulae to calculate a 'least-squares' linear regression equation;
- interpret the regression equation in the context of the problem given;
- find and interpret the coefficient of determination R^2; and
- find and interpret the standard error of the estimate.

The linear regression model

Scatterplots and correlation coefficients show us whether or not two variables have a strong linear relationship. Correlation coefficients are used to describe the strength and direction of a linear relationship that may exist between two variables, but regression analysis calculates the equation of the straight line which best models the relationship. Not all relationships between variables will be linear, so the initial exploratory work with the scatterplots is most important in order to determine whether or not a linear model is appropriate. If the data cannot be approximated using a linear model, a suitable non-linear model should be chosen, or the data may be transformed to produce a linear relationship. Some of the more common transformations include square roots, reciprocals and logarithms.

In this book we will consider only simple linear regression models involving two variables — an independent variable, usually denoted by X and the dependent variable, usually denoted by Y. We are primarily interested in predicting values of the dependent variable given specific values of the independent variable.

Once we know the equation of the straight line we can predict values of the dependent variable, given values of the independent variable. For example, consider the time spent recovering in hospital after surgery for patients of various ages. The following data were collected from 10 cases involving knee surgery, and a scatterplot constructed for the data. The plot is used in deciding whether a straight line can adequately describe the data; from the plot of this data it seems reasonable to use a linear model to describe the data.

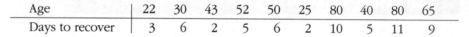

Age	22	30	43	52	50	25	80	40	80	65
Days to recover	3	6	2	5	6	2	10	5	11	9

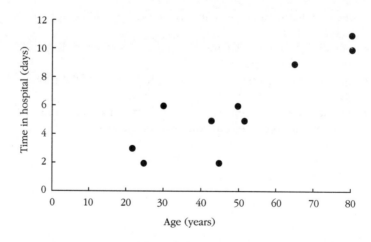

Figure 8.1   Scatterplot of sample data (time spent in hospital after surgery vs age).

The scatterplot for the data shows clearly that, on average, younger people need less time in hospital following surgery than older people. It would be useful, however, to be able to predict how long patients, on average, will need hospital care after surgery. If we draw a straight line through the middle of the cloud of

Practical statistics for the health sciences

points in the scatterplot, averaging out those points above and below the line, then we would have a type of average prediction model. While it is not possible to find a straight line that will pass through every data point, it is possible to find the line that will best fit the data points. This is achieved by a process known as the method of least squares.

The resulting straight line is known as the *line of best fit* because its position among the points minimises the variation of the points above and below the line. The line of best fit has been included on the scatterplot of the same data points in Figure 8.2.

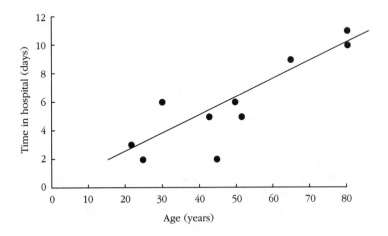

Figure 8.2 Line of best fit for the scatterplot in Figure 8.1.

Once the equation of the line of best fit has been established it can be used to estimate or predict values of the dependent variable. In our example the dependent variable is the number of days spent in hospital after surgery, because that is what is affected by a patient's age. (It would not make sense to say that a patient's age depended upon the amount of time spent in hospital after surgery.)

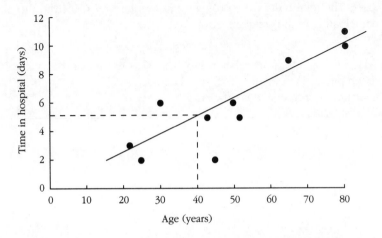

Figure 8.3 Predicting the value of the dependent variable (time in hospital) using the line of best fit.

Once the position of the line of best fit is known we can use it to make predictions about the length of hospital stay following surgery given a patient's age. For example, Figure 8.3 shows the length of stay expected for a 40-year-old patient is about 5 days. Without the equation for the straight line we can only obtain an approximation from the graph. To be more precise in our estimate we would need to use a *regression equation*.

The regression equation

The equation of a straight line involves expressing the relationship between the dependent variable Y in terms of an independent variable X. In our example we would express the relationship between the expected length of stay in hospital after surgery (Y) in terms of a patient's age (X). There are many ways of writing equations for straight lines, but the most common patterns are

$$y = mx + c, \quad ax + by = c$$

Any equation for a straight line can be transformed to fit the form $y = mx + c$ or $y = c + mx$. When we use this pattern in the context of linear regression it is common to use the notation

$$\hat{y} = b_0 + b_1 x$$

In this equation $\hat{y}$ represents the estimated or predicted value of y, and x represents the independent variable. The values b_0 and b_1 are often referred to as the *regression coefficients*. When x is zero $\hat{y}$ will be equal to b_0, so that when the line is plotted it will intercept the y-axis at the point b_0 (called the *y-intercept*). The coefficient b_1 represents the *slope* or *gradient* of the line; that is, the average amount of change that occurs in y for each one unit change in x. The coefficient b_1 may be either positive or negative, depending upon the direction of the change in y as the variable x increases. In our example we see that there is a positive relationship; that is as x increases so does y. Example 8.1 looks at plotting a given regression line and interpreting the regression coefficients in the context of a particular situation.

EXAMPLE   **8.1**

A first-aid training program was recently introduced by the managers of a local industrial complex. The total cost of the program (y) was linearly related to the number of employees (x) participating in the program by the regression equation

$$\hat{y} = 2550 + 750x$$

(a) Sketch the graph of the relationship and use it to predict the total costs to the company if six employees undertake the first-aid course.
(b) Interpret the regression coefficients.

Practical statistics for the health sciences

EXAMPLE 8.1 cont.

Solution

(a) The graph of $\hat{y} = 2550 + 750x$ is constructed by substituting several values for x into the equation and calculating the corresponding $\hat{y}$ values. The points are plotted and joined by a straight line.

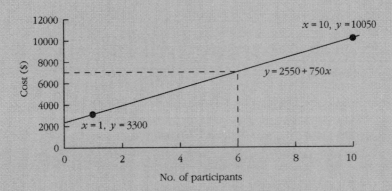

From the graph, if six employees undertook the first-aid course the total cost to the company would be about $7000. Using the equation to predict for $x = 6$ gives

$$\hat{y} = 2550 + (750 \times 6) = 2550 + 4500 = 7050$$

(b) The line in the graph has a slope (gradient) of 750, and a y-intercept of 2550. A slope of +750 means that as x increases by one, $\hat{y}$ will increase by 750. In other words, each additional employee will add $750 to the total cost. The graph intersects the y-axis at $y = \$2550$ indicating that even without any employees involved in the program the total costs will still be $2550! This could be seen as the *overheads* or *fixed costs*.

Determining the mathematical equation

The regression line is positioned such that the squared differences between the data points and the line itself are minimised. The equation for the line is thus sometimes called the *least squares regression equation*. (The calculation of the standard deviation uses the same concept except that squared deviations from the *mean* are minimised.) The values of the coefficients b_0 and b_1 for the regression line $\hat{y} = b_0 + b_1 x$ that best fits the data points (sample size = n) can be found using the following formulae:

$$b_1 = \frac{n \sum xy - \sum x \sum y}{n \sum x^2 - (\sum x)^2} \text{ and } b_0 = \bar{y} - b_1 \bar{x}$$

These formulae make use of the raw scores comprising the data set. In Example 8.2 we will find the equation of the straight line that best fits the hospital stay data. In this case the age of the patient is the independent (control) variable and the days spent in hospital recovering is the dependent (response) variable. We are interested in predicting the recovery period of a patient given their age, and to do this we require a formula of the form $\hat{y} = b_0 + b_1 x$ where $\hat{y}$ represents the predicted time in hospital.

EXAMPLE 8.2

The time spent recovering in hospital after knee surgery for 10 patients of various ages is given below. Find the regression equation for this data and use it to predict the expected length of hospital stay for a 40-year-old patient after knee surgery.

Age (X)	22	30	43	52	50	25	80	40	80	65
Days in Hospital	3	6	2	5	6	2	10	5	11	9

Solution

From the above data,

$$\Sigma x = 487, \quad \Sigma y = 59, \quad \Sigma xy = 3407, \quad (\Sigma x)^2 = 237169, \quad \Sigma x^2 = 27687, \quad n = 10$$

Substituting into the respective formulae for b_1 and b_0, we get

$$b_1 = \frac{10 \times 3407 - 487 \times 59}{10 \times 27687 - 237169} = \frac{34070 - 28733}{39701} = 0.13443$$

$$b_0 = \frac{59}{10} - (0.13443)\frac{487}{10} = 5.9 - 6.548 = -0.648$$

Therefore the regression equation is $\hat{y} = -0.65 + 0.134x$.

For a 40-year-old patient the predicted time is

$$\hat{y} = -0.65 + 0.134(40) = 4.71 \text{ days.}$$

The same result is easily obtained from Minitab using the REGRESS command as shown in the abbreviated Minitab printout in Figure 8.3. Note that in using this command you are required to specify the dependent variable first, followed by the number of independent variables being used in the model, and finally the independent variable(s). In this case only one independent variable is being used in the model to predict hospital stay.

```
MTB > regr c2 1 c1

The regression equation is
Recovery = - 0.65 + 0.134 Age

Predictor     Coef     Stdev   t-ratio      p
Constant    -0.647     1.358     -0.48   0.647
Age        0.13443   0.02581      5.21   0.000

s = 1.626     R-sq = 77.2%    R-sq(adj) = 74.4%
```

Figure 8.3 Minitab printout for regression of hospital recovery upon age.

The interpretation proceeds as follows. For patients between the ages of 22 and 80, an increase of one year in age is likely to add 0.134 days to hospital recovery time after knee surgery. So for a 10-year difference in ages you could expect a patient to spend an extra 1.34 days in hospital recovering. The interpretation of the coefficient $b_0 = -0.65$ is not quite as straightforward. This is the predicted stay in hospital when age equals zero. In the context of this example a length of stay in hospital of −0.65 days has no sensible meaning — it is simply the regression constant for this particular model. It may also indicate that if the age range were to be extended to include younger patients the linear model may no longer be appropriate. This can be seen in Figure 8.4 which is based upon a larger data set than that used above. The age range has been increased to include some younger patients.

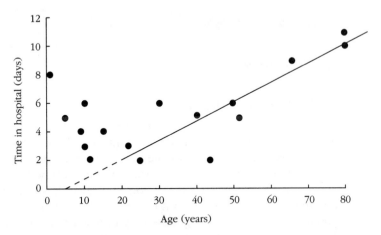

Figure 8.4 The danger in extrapolating beyond the range of sampled data is that the same relationship may not exist.

The scatterplot above highlights the important point that when using a regression model for prediction purposes we should only consider the *relevant range* of the independent variable. In other words we should not use the model for prediction purposes involving ages of patients that lie outside the range of the data originally used to generate the model, in this case ages between 22 and 80. We may *interpolate*, but not *extrapolate*, because the assumed linear relationship may not hold over a wider range of ages.

The actual length of stay for any age group will vary, but it will tend to be centred around the value predicted by the regression equation. In this sense the regression equation is only modelling the situation by describing an *average* relationship between length of stay and age. Obviously, variables other than age will play a role in determining how long a patient stays in hospital after surgery.

8.2   Determining the suitability of the model

Two questions that often arise from a regression analysis are 'How accurate are the various regression estimates?' and 'How good is the model?'

The easiest way to answer these questions is to reconsider the Minitab printout for the hospital stay example reproduced in Figure 8.5 with two statistics highlighted in bold type. These two statistics are an indication of just how good the linear model actually is.

```
MTB > regr c2 1 c1

The regression equation is
Recovery = - 0.65 + 0.134 Age

Predictor     Coef      Stdev    t-ratio       p
Constant     -0.647     1.358      -0.48    0.647
Age          0.13443    0.02581     5.21    0.000

s = 1.626    R-sq = 77.2%    R-sq(adj) = 74.4%
```

Figure 8.5 Minitab printout for the hospital stay example.

The coefficient of determination (R^2)

From the Minitab printout in Figure 8.5 we see that the R^2-value is 77.2%. This means that the regression model accounts for 77.2% of the variation in length of hospital stay by using the variable *age* as the predictor. In other words 77.2% of the variation in length of hospital stay can be explained by variation in age. This implies then, that 22.8% of the variation in length of hospital stay has to be explained by other factors. At this point it becomes a little subjective as to whether or not you feel that the model is good enough for your prediction purposes. There are no hard and fast rules for accepting and therefore using a model. The variation that is not explained by the model (ie $100 - R^2$) is often the deciding factor. For the above case we think that the model is quite reasonable, given that more than three quarters of the variation in hospital stay can be explained by a patient's age.

We now have two ways of predicting a variable Y:

(a) we can use the *mean* ($\bar{y}$) or

(b) we can use the regression equation ($\hat{y} = b_0 + b_1 x$).

In order to determine which is the better predictor, we consider the sum of the squared deviations of the actual y-values from their predicted values. For method (a) this means finding the sum of the squared deviations of the y-values about the mean $\bar{y}$. We write this as $\Sigma(y - \bar{y})^2$ and define it to be the *total sum of squares* (*SST*). On the other hand, if we now calculate the squared deviations of the actual y-values from those predicted by the regression model (method (b)), then we obtain $\Sigma(y - \hat{y})^2$, known as the *error sum of squares* (*SSE*). If these quantities are actually calculated for the length of hospital stay data, we get the following values:

$$\Sigma(y - \bar{y})^2 = 92.90 \qquad \text{and} \qquad \Sigma(y - \hat{y})^2 = 21.155$$

Obviously, the squared deviations of the y-values about the regression line (represented by $\hat{y}$) are considerably less than those measured about the mean. Using the regression line resulted in a considerable reduction in the total squared error. This reduction is found by subtracting one from the other as follows:

$$\Sigma(y - \bar{y})^2 - \Sigma(y - \hat{y})^2 = 92.90 - 21.155 = 71.745$$

The resulting reduction is defined as the *regression sum of squares* (*SSR*). If we consider this reduction in percentage terms, with respect to the squared deviations about the mean (92.90) then we get

Practical statistics for the health sciences

$$\text{percentage reduction} = \frac{71.745}{92.90} \times 100 = 77.228$$

This value is the same as the R^2-value given above. Therefore the percentage reduction in the total squared error obtained by using the regression line rather than the mean is the same as the *coefficient of determination*. Hence, we can define R^2 as:

$$R^2 = \frac{SST - SSE}{SST}$$

As we have seen, the variation of points around the mean $\bar{y}$ is called the total variation (SST). The vertical deviations of the y-scores around the regression line are called the *unexplained* variation (SSE) because they cannot be explained by the value of x alone. There is *still* dispersion even after the line is taken into account. The amount of deviation explained by the regression line is the difference between the total variation and the unexplained variation.

explained variation = total variation – unexplained variation
$\quad\quad SSR \quad\quad\quad = \quad\quad SST \quad\quad - \quad\quad\quad SSE$

(a) Scatter around mean length of hospital stay

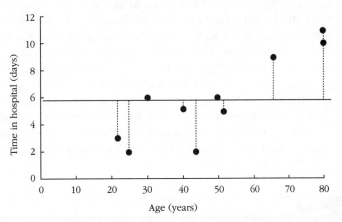

(b) Scatter around regression line

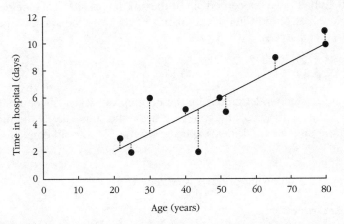

Figure 8.6 A comparison of the scatter of scores around the regression line with scatter around the mean *y* indicates the extent to which predictions based on the line are superior to those based upon the mean.

The percentage of explained variation is the ratio of the explained variation to the total variation.

$$\text{percentage of explained variation} = \frac{\text{explained variation}}{\text{total variation}}$$

$$\text{or } R^2 = \frac{SSR}{SST} = \frac{SST - SSE}{SST}$$

The coefficient of determination (R^2) is simply the square of the correlation coefficient.

The standard error of the estimate (S_e)

The squared deviations of the sample observations from the regression line are used in calculating a *standard error*. This standard error of estimate can be thought of as simply a standard deviation which uses the regression line as a reference point, rather than the mean. It is defined as

$$S_e = \sqrt{\frac{\Sigma(y - \hat{y})^2}{n - 2}} = \sqrt{\frac{SSE}{n - 2}}$$

So S_e, the standard error of the estimate, is a measure of the scatter of the sample observations around the regression line. It is a measure of the prediction error, and for the hospital stay example we have $S_e = 1.626$. This represents the standard deviation of the sample observations around the regression line.

Example 8.3 makes use of the Minitab regression output. Initially the data were put into columns one and two, and named accordingly. To have completed the regression analysis by hand would have required considerably more effort, as the calculations of the regression coefficients b_0 and b_1, the R^2-value and S_e are tedious. This example is one in which there is a inverse relationship between the two variables; that is, as one variable increases in value the other decreases. This gives rise to a negative correlation coefficient as well as a negative gradient (b_1-value) for the regression line.

EXAMPLE 8.3

The following data was collected from a sample of workers at a city factory site. For some time management had been concerned about the amount of sick-leave being taken by employees. The two variables of most interest to management were the age and the number of sick-days taken by the employees.

Age	27	61	37	23	46	58	29	36	64	40
Sickies	15	6	10	18	9	7	14	11	5	8

(a) Find a regression model predicting the number of 'sickies' given the age of an employee.
(b) Interpret the coefficients, and comment upon the suitability of the model.
(c) Predict the number of 'sickies' expected from a 50-year-old employee.

Solution
From Minitab the following printout is obtained:

```
MTB > plot c2 c1
```

EXAMPLE 8.3   cont.

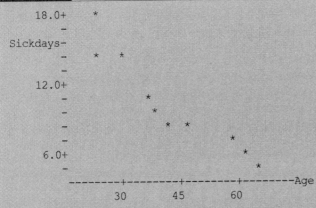

```
MTB > correlate c2 c1

Correlation of Sickdays and Age = -0.934
```

The scatterplot of the data suggests that a linear model is appropriate, and this is supported by the strong negative correlation coefficient of – 0.934. The regression printout from Minitab follows:

```
MTB > regress c2 1 c1;
SUBC> predict 50.

The regression equation is
Sickdays = 21.0 - 0.257 Age

Predictor     Coef      Stdev     t-ratio      p
Constant    21.000      1.535      13.68     0.000
Age        -0.25720    0.03484     -7.38     0.000

s = 1.600    R-sq = 87.2%    R-sq(adj) = 85.6%

Analysis of Variance

SOURCE       DF        SS        MS        F        p
Regression    1     139.61    139.61    54.51    0.000
Error         8      20.49      2.56
Total         9     160.10

Unusual Observations
Obs.   Age   Sickdays      Fit    Stdev.Fit    Residual    St.Resid
  4   23.0     18.000   15.084       0.822       2.916       2.12R
```

R denotes an obs. with a large st. resid.

```
   Fit    Stdev.Fit       95% C.I.            95% P.I.
  8.139      0.585    ( 6.791, 9.488)    ( 4.209, 12.070)
```

(a) From the printout the regression equation is Sickdays = 21 – 0.257 (Age).

EXAMPLE **8.3** **cont.**

(b) From the equation, $b_0 = 21$, and $b_1 = -0.257$. Interpretation of $b_0 = 21$ is meaningless because an employee cannot be zero years of age. The value $b_1 = -0.257$ implies that for each extra year of age an employee will take 0.257 sick-leave days less per year. That is, on average, a 40-year-old employee will take 2.57 sickdays fewer than a 30-year-old employee.

    The model has an R^2-value of 87.2% or 0.8720. This means that 87.2% of the variation in sick-leave days can be explained by the age of the employee. In other words the model explains 87.2% of the variation in sick-leave. This is quite a strong model. The standard error S_e is given on the printout as $s = 1.600$. This means that employees' sick-leave days can be expected to vary around the regression line by ± 1.600 days, on average. This seems to be reasonable given the nature of the data.

(c) By substituting the value Age = 50 into the regression equation we get the predicted number of sick-leave days for a 50-year-old employee as 8.139 days.

    As a further point of interest, the correlation between these two variables is given by the square root of the R^2-value. So, we have $r = \sqrt{R^2} = \sqrt{0.872} = -0.934$. Note the use of the negative sign because of the negative relationship between these two variables.

8.3   *Analysis of the residuals*

The residuals consist of the differences between the actual y-values and those predicted by the model. That is,

$$\text{residual} = (y - \hat{y})$$

It is important to analyse the residuals of any regression model when considering the appropriateness of the model. If the model is reasonable we expect the residuals to:

- average zero,
- be normally distributed, and
- occur randomly with respect to the values of the independent variable.

If any of the above conditions are not satisfied then the model may not be appropriate.

It is beyond the scope of this introductory text to fully discuss residual analysis, except to say that the Minitab commands DESCRIBE, HISTOGRAM and PLOT can be used to investigate the three points mentioned above, depending on which column is used to store the residuals. The command REGRESS c2 1 c1 c3 will generate a regression model for data in columns 2 (dependent variable) and 1 (independent variable), and at the same time store the standardised residuals from the model in column 3.

1 Given the following set of paired X and Y scores, answer the questions below.

X	7	10	9	13	7	11	13
Y	1	2	4	3	3	4	5

(a) Construct a scatterplot of the paired scores.
(b) Determine the least squares regression line for Y given X.
(c) Determine the least squares regression line for X given Y. Are they the same? Explain.
(d) Draw both regression lines on the scatterplot and determine their point of intersection.
(e) What value would you predict for Y given $X = 12$?

2 An instructor conducts a study to investigate the relationship between anxiety and the performance of nursing students in a test of procedures involving emergency cases. Ten students are chosen at random and, prior to their test, are given an anxiety questionnaire. The final test results and the respective anxiety scores for the 10 nurses were:

Anxiety	28	41	35	39	31	42	50	46	45	37
Test score	82	58	63	89	92	64	55	70	51	72

(a) Construct a scatter plot of the paired scores using *anxiety* as the X variable. .
(b) Determine the least squares regression line for predicting the test score given the anxiety level. Should b_1 be positive or negative? Why?
(c) Interpret the coefficients b_0 and b_1.
(d) If a student has an anxiety score of 38, what value would you predict for her test score?
(e) Calculate the value of R^2. How do you interpret this value?

3 The manager of a large medical supplies store has recently started a nation-wide advertising campaign. Records of monthly advertising costs and profits are shown below, in thousands of dollars.

	Jan	Feb	Mar	Apr	May	Jun	Jul
Cost	10.0	14.0	11.4	15.6	16.8	11.2	13.2
Profit	125	200	160	150	210	110	125

(a) Derive the least squares regression line for predicting monthly profits from monthly advertising costs.

(b) In August the manager plans to spend $17000 on advertising. Based upon the above data how much profit should he expect that month?
(c) Given the relationship shown by the data, why should the manager not spend a lot more money on advertising?

4 For the following pairs of observations, X is the intensity of a sound stimulus and Y is the time taken by a patient to respond to the stimulus.

X	Y	X	Y	X	Y
1.3	1.70	2.1	1.62	2.4	1.48
3.0	1.00	3.8	1.19	4.5	1.23
5.1	0.80	5.7	0.59	6.0	0.35
6.2	0.61	6.9	0.70	7.4	0.44
7.4	0.31	8.1	0.33	9.6	0.30
10.0	0.18	10.9	0.15		

Use the Minitab printout below to answer the following questions.
(a) Determine the equation to the least squares regression line. Sketch the line onto the scatterplot.
(b) Interpret the regression coefficients in the context of the problem.
(c) How much variation in response time can be explained by variation in the intensity of the sound stimulus?
(d) Determine the standard error of the estimate and explain what it means.
(e) Predict the average time to react to a sound stimulus of intensity of 12.0. How do you explain this result?

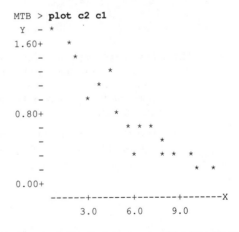

```
MTB > plot c2 c1
   Y  - *
  1.60+     *
     -        *
     -            *
     -          *
     -       *
  0.80+     *
     -            *
     -           * * *
     -                 *
     -          *    * * *
     -                   * *
  0.00+
     ------+-------+-------+------X
          3.0     6.0     9.0
```

```
MTB > regr c2 1 c1
The regression equation is
Y = 1.76 - 0.168 X

Predictor   Coef    Stdev    t-ratio      p
Constant    1.7571  0.1129    15.57    0.000
X          -0.16824 0.01731   -9.72    0.000

s = 0.1968  R-sq = 86.3% R-sq(adj) = 85.4%
```

5 What is the equation of a straight line with the following characteristics:

(a) slope of 10.2 and y-intercept of 5?

(b) slope of 55 and y-intercept of 0?

(c) $b_0 = 27$, $b_1 = -2$?

(d) $b_0 = 4$, $b_1 = 0$?

6 The printout below shows the regression output for predicting nursing theory test scores from test scores based upon clinical practice. From the printout, determine the following:

(a) The regression equation;

(b) The coefficient of determination;

(c) The standard error of the estimate;

(d) Given a clinical practice mark of 50, what does the model predict the theory test score will be? How reliable is this prediction?

```
MTB > regr c2 1 c1
The regression equation is
Theory = 22.5 + 0.755 Prac

Predictor   Coef    Stdev    t-ratio
Constant    22.47   10.22     2.20
Prac        0.7546  0.1417    5.32

s = 11.51  R-sq = 49.4%  R-sq(adj) = 47.7%
```

7 The following data represent the results of a study for which X is the quantity of a food supplement in the diet of chickens, and Y is a measurement of the hardness of the eggshells laid by the chickens.

X	0.12	0.21	0.28	0.34	0.15	0.48	0.61
Y	0.70	0.98	1.04	1.16	0.78	1.40	1.75

X	0.42	0.13	0.10	0.19	0.21	0.26	0.34
Y	1.31	0.76	0.65	0.90	0.95	1.10	1.24

X	0.51	0.71	0.68	0.62	0.17
Y	1.51	1.95	1.83	1.75	0.82

(a) Obtain a scatterplot of the data points and comment on the suitability or otherwise of using a linear regression model to predict eggshell hardness, given the amount of food supplement in the diet of chickens.

(b) The regression line is to be used only if at least 90% of the variation in hardness can be explained by variation in the amount of food supplement. Should the line be used? If so, estimate the average shell hardness that would occur with 0.50 unit of the food supplement in the diet.

8 The following data give the time taken for ulcers of various sizes to heal.

Radius of ulcer (mm)	Time of healing (weeks)
2.4	1.5
2.8	4.3
5.6	7.8
2.7	2.4
8.6	10.3
3.5	4.9
6.6	5.9
3.4	2.1
8.4	7.3
5.7	6.1

(a) Perform a regression analysis on the data, commenting on the suitability of a linear model to predict the healing time of ulcers.

(b) What effect would an increase of 1 mm in the radius of an ulcer have on the healing time predicted by the model?

(c) How do you interpret the regression constant for this case?

(d) Would you be justified in using the model to predict the healing time for an ulcer of radius 15 mm? Explain.

Progress review 3

1 (a) For the following data the variable X represents the age (in years) of 5 vehicles and Y represents the total distance (in thousands of kilometres) travelled by those vehicles.

X	3	2	5	7	10
Y	50	40	95	145	180

The summary statistics are:

$\bar{X} = 5.4$, $\bar{Y} = 102$, $\sum X^2 = 187$, $\sum Y^2 = 66550$, $\sum X.Y = 3520$

Use the information above to find the regression equation for the data and use it to predict the total distance travelled by a 6-year-old vehicle.

(b) Use the Minitab printout below for the vehicle data in part (a) to answer the following questions.
   (i) What proportion of the variation in total distance travelled can be explained by the variation in the age of the vehicle?
   (ii) What is the standard error of the estimate?
   (iii) Comment on the overall suitability of the regression model.
   (iv) In any given year, how many kilometres would you expect a vehicle to travel?

```
MTB > regr c2 1 c1

The regression equation is
distance = 1.60 + 18.6 age


Predictor    Coef     Stdev     t-ratio        p
Constant     1.602    9.341        0.17     0.875
age         18.592    1.527       12.17     0.001


s = 9.804   R-sq = 98.0%   R-sq(adj) = 97.4%


Analysis of Variance

SOURCE        DF        SS        MS         F        p
Regression     1     14242     14242    148.17     0.001
Error          3       288        96
Total          4     14530
```

2 A test is given to a sample of eight students (A to H) and each student is given a mark out of 50. Each student is also ranked by the tutor with regard to knowledge of the same material included in the test. A ranking of 1 indicates a low level of knowledge. The results for each student are shown below:

Result	A	B	C	D	E	F	G	H
Test score	40	25	45	30	48	30	50	45
Tutor's ranking	5	2	4	1	8	3	7	6

Find the correlation between the tutor's rankings of these students and their test scores.

CHAPTER OUTLINE

9.1 Sampling distributions
Interpreting varying sample statistics using sampling distributions.

9.2 The Central Limit Theorem
The theorem and its importance. The Central Limit Theorem is empirically rather than theoretically justified. The standard error of the mean, and the corrections required if sampling from a finite population.

9.3 Estimation
Point estimates and interval estimates. How to calculate confidence intervals using formulae and using Minitab.

9.4 Estimation error
The meaning of the width of the confidence interval in real problems and how this may be restricted.

9.5 Estimating sample size
How large must samples be if we wish to restrict the level of confidence or the size of the error?

9.6 Dealing with small samples
The t-distribution and its use.

9.7 Using Minitab to obtain t-intervals
The tint command.

CHAPTER NINE

Estimation

LEARNING OBJECTIVES

After reading this chapter you should be able to:

- apply the Central Limit Theorem to find the probability of the occurrence in given intervals of various sample means;
- calculate and interpret the standard error of the mean;
- make appropriate use of the finite population correction factor;
- find point estimates for population parameters;
- calculate interval estimates for the population mean given sample data and a specified level of required confidence;
- calculate the error involved in the estimation of the mean;
- given a required level of confidence and a limited error tolerance, calculate the size of the sample needed for the estimate;
- recognise when the distribution of sample means may be expected to follow a normal distribution and when it would be better modelled by Student's t-distribution. Correctly use appropriate statistical tables.

9.1   *Sampling distributions*

Collecting data from a whole population is usually prohibitively expensive, both in terms of time and cost. It is also impractical, especially in quality control where measures such as strength and durability must be measured by testing items to the point of destruction. Researchers must be satisfied with collecting data from samples and using statistics calculated from them to estimate corresponding population parameters.

Sample statistics, like the mean and the variance, vary from sample to sample. Consider the following situation, for example. Internal parasites can be a life-threatening problem for children in third-world countries. A community health worker who wanted to attract international aid to improve water quality in her region wished to establish the incidence of parasites in weaned children under the age of 5 years. Cleaning out the parasites and counting them was indeed a difficult procedure to monitor, and funding for this research was limited. It was decided to study just 25 children. Clearly the group selected would not be identical to any other such group selected. Each sample would be different, and the mean and the standard deviation for the number of parasites would vary from sample to sample.

You can take 100 samples of the same size from the same population and obtain 100 different sample results, all supposedly measuring the same variable. Fortunately there are known patterns for the distributions of sample statistics like the mean and the standard deviation. Knowledge of these patterns enables the researcher to make generalisations about the population based on the statistics from just one sample. This phenomenon is seen in the differences that occur in the findings of the various political polls that are taken, particularly around election times.

We are primarily interested in the distribution of the sample statistic. This distribution is based upon all possible samples of size n from a given population and consists of a list of all possible values that the statistic can take and their associated probabilities.

9.2   *The Central Limit Theorem*

The Central Limit Theorem is the basis for many of the generalisations we are able to make in statistics. Although it may be proven mathematically, we shall only state the properties of the theorem and illustrate these properties using a Minitab simulation.

If all possible samples, of size n, are taken from any population with a mean μ and standard deviation σ, the distribution of the sample means will have the following characteristics:

(a) The *mean of the sample means* will be the same as the population mean
$$\mu_{\bar{x}} = \mu,$$

(b) The *variance of the sample means* will be equal to the population variance divided by the sample size. We write this as

$$\sigma_{\bar{x}}^2 = \frac{\sigma^2}{n}, \text{ which implies that } \sigma_{\bar{x}} = \frac{\sigma}{\sqrt{n}}$$

    Practical statistics for the health sciences

(c) The sample mean, $\bar{x}$, will be *normally distributed* when the population is normal, or will be approximately normally distributed for samples of size 30 or more when the parent population is not normally distributed. The approximation to normality improves as the sample size increases.

To illustrate the last point, we can use Minitab to simulate the drawing of 150 samples from a given population for which the parameters μ and σ are known. The sample sizes considered included $n = 2$, $n = 5$, $n = 15$, and $n = 30$. The effects of increasing the sample size upon the distribution of each group of 150 sample means can be seen in the dotplots and the descriptive statistics obtained from Minitab.

```
MTB > dotplot c1

Each dot represents 6 points

             .
            :.
          .:::::
         ::::::...
         ::::::::.  .
         ::::::::::::
        :::::::::::::::.:........
      -+---------+---------+---------+--------Popn
      0.0       8.0      16.0      24.0      32.0
```

Figure 9.1 Dotplot of population from which the samples in Figure 9.2 were taken.

The dotplot in Figure 9.1 represents the population from which the samples in Figure 9.2 were taken. It is clear that the population is not normal, for it is considerably skewed to the right (positively skewed). The mean and standard deviation for the defined population are $\mu = 4$ and $\sigma = 4$. So according to the Central Limit Theorem the mean of the sample means should be 4 and the standard deviation of the sample means should be $\frac{4}{\sqrt{n}}$. In fact, because Minitab is simulating the process we can only hope to get results *close* to those expected.

The shapes of the dotplots below clearly show that, as the sample size increases from $n = 2$ to $n = 30$, the distribution of the sample means appears to become '*more normal*' and considerably less spread out. The descriptive statistics for each group of sample means shows that, as n increases, the mean of the sample means gets closer to the value of the population mean ($\mu = 4$). The standard deviations show that, as n increases, the variability of the sample means decreases. Notice also how the median approaches the mean as n increases. This emphasises the underlying symmetry of the distribution of sample means as the sample size increases.

```
                .:
              :  ::
             ::  ::. .
             ::  ::: :
            :::::::: :. :
           .::::::: :: .:
           :::::::::.:::.::
          ::::::::::::::::::::....:: ::. ..   : .
         -+----------+----------+----------+--------n=2
                  .
                  :
                  :
               . :
              ::: :
              ::: ::..: .
             .::: :::: :
             :::::::::: :
             :::::::::: :.
             ::::::::::: :
             ::::::::::::.:: ::..:      ..
          -+----------+----------+----------+--------n=5
                . :
                : :
               .:.:
               :::::
              .:::::
               :::::
               :::::
              .:::::
               :::::
             .::::::::::::: :
             ::::::::::::::.:
          -+----------+----------+----------+--------n=15
Each dot represents 2 points
                  .
                  :
                . :.
               :.:::
               :::::
               :::::
               :::::
               :::::
              ::::::..
             .::::::::::..
          -+----------+----------+----------+--------n=30
         0.0        4.0        8.0       12.0      16.0


MTB > desc c32 - c35


             N      MEAN     MEDIAN     TRMEAN     STDEV
   n=2      150     3.643     2.876      3.379      2.708
   n=5      150     3.882     3.605      3.728      1.840
   n=15     150     4.0945    3.9521     4.0531     1.1889
   n=30     150     4.0339    4.0284     4.0050     0.8367
```

Figure 9.2 Dotplots of samples drawn from population in Figure 9.1.

In order to calculate probabilities associated with specific sample means, we follow the usual procedure of using the standard normal distribution. In particular, we have

$$z = \frac{\bar{x} - \mu}{\sigma_{\bar{x}}}$$

This formula can be used only if we know the actual population standard deviation. If σ is not known, which is usually the case, then we have to use the best estimate we have, which is the sample standard deviation, s. In this case we have $s_{\bar{x}}$ being used to approximate $\sigma_{\bar{x}}$, where $s_{\bar{x}}$ is defined as

$$s_{\bar{x}} = \frac{s}{\sqrt{n}}$$

This approximation is quite good for $n \geq 30$, so we have

$$z = \frac{\bar{x} - \mu}{s_{\bar{x}}}$$

Standard error of the mean, $\sigma_{\bar{x}}$

Each sample mean is an estimate of the true mean, and the variability of sample means is described by the *standard error of the mean*, defined as $\sigma_{\bar{x}}$; that is, the standard deviation of the sample means. Variability between sample means will occur due to random differences in samples arising as a result of two factors: (a) variation in the original population, and (b) variation in sample size. The standard error of the mean is best approximated by $s_{\bar{x}}$ when σ is unknown.

The Central Limit Theorem is important in statistical theory because it enables us to utilise the mathematical properties of the normal distribution when analysing the sample mean, $\bar{x}$. This is despite the fact that the original distribution of the population may well be not normal or may even be unknown. Knowing that sample means are normally distributed for large samples allows us to determine probabilities associated with particular sample means, which in turn enables us to define levels of significance for samples of various sizes. You may find some of the probabilities in Example 9.1 quite surprising, but recall that sample means do not vary as much as individual values. For the example below the variation of individual values is given by $\sigma = 6$, whereas the variation of the sample means is given by $\sigma_{\bar{x}} = 0.937$.

EXAMPLE 9.1

The heart rates of students studying Physical Education are typically less than those for students in other courses. The average heart rate for all Physical Education students is believed to be 65 beats per minute with a standard deviation of 6 beats per minute. A random sample of 41 students is chosen. Calculate the probability that
(a) the sample mean will be less than 62,
(b) the sample mean will be more than 70,
(c) the sample mean will be between 62 and 68.
Solution
From the information given we have the following summary:

$$\mu = 65, \; \sigma = 6, \; n = 41, \text{ so } \sigma_{\bar{x}} = \frac{6}{\sqrt{41}} = 0.937$$

EXAMPLE 9.1

cont.

(a) For $\bar{x} = 62$, $z = \dfrac{62 - 65}{0.937} = -3.20$, and $Pr(z \le -3.2) = 0.5 - 0.4993 = 0.0007$

Therefore it is not likely that a sample of 41 will have a mean ≤ 62 (Pr = 0.0007).

(b) For $\bar{x} = 70$, $z = \dfrac{70 - 65}{0.937} = 5.34$, and $Pr(z \ge 5.34) = 0.5 - 0.5 = 0.00$

Correct to four decimal places, the probability that a sample of 41 will have a sample mean ≥ 70 is zero.

(c) From part (a), the probability that $\bar{x}$ lies between 62 and 65 is 0.4993. As the normal distribution is symmetrical, this is the same as the probability that $\bar{x}$ lies between 65 and 68. Therefore the probability that $\bar{x}$ lies between 62 and 68 is 0.9986. In other words, if the above values for μ and σ are correct then there is a 99.86% chance that a sample of 41 will have a mean between 62 and 68.

Sampling from a finite population

If the sample size is small relative to the size of the population ($n \le 5\%$ of N) then sampling *without replacement* yields essentially the same variability among samples as does sampling *with replacement*. However, if the sample size is more than 5% of the population the variability occurring as a result of sampling without replacement will be somewhat different from that arising from sampling with replacement. This difference occurs because the probabilities of selecting particular items *change* if sampling is done without replacement.

To compensate for sampling without replacement, the standard error of the mean is modifed to reflect the changing probabilities. This adjustment, however, is only necessary if the sample size is more than 5% of the population. The amount by which the standard error of the mean is modified is called the *finite population correction factor*, and it reflects the proportion of observations that have not been included in the sample. This correction factor is defined as $\sqrt{\frac{N-n}{N}}$. The standard error of the mean is multiplied by this correction factor when the sample size, n, is more than 5% of the population, N. Hence the adjusted formula for calculating $\sigma_{\bar{x}}$ when $n > 5\%$ of N is

$$\sigma_{\bar{x}} = \frac{\sigma}{\sqrt{n}} \cdot \sqrt{\frac{N-n}{N}}$$

EXAMPLE 9.2

The heart rates of students studying Physical Education are typically less than those for students in other courses. The average heart rate for all Physical Education students is believed to be 65 beats per minute with a standard deviation of 6 beats per minute. A random sample of 41 students is chosen from the 225 students currently enrolled. Find the probability that the sample mean will be between 62 and 68.

EXAMPLE   9.2   cont.

Solution
From the information given,

$$\mu = 65, \sigma = 6, n = 41, N = 225$$

As n is more than 5% of $N(\frac{41}{225} = 0.1822)$ the correction factor should be used

$$\text{ie } \sigma_{\bar{x}} = \frac{\sigma}{\sqrt{n}} \cdot \sqrt{\frac{N-n}{N}} = \frac{6}{\sqrt{41}} \cdot \sqrt{\frac{225-41}{225}}$$

$$\sigma_{\bar{x}} = 0.937 \times 0.9043 = 0.8473$$

For $\bar{x} = 62$, $z = \frac{62-65}{0.8473} = -3.54$, and $\Pr(-3.54 \le z \le 0) = 0.4998$

The result for $\bar{x} = 68$ is the same (symmetry of the normal curve), so the probability that the sample mean will lie between 62 and 68 is $2 \times 0.4998 = 0.9996$. This value is slightly different to that obtained in part (c) of Example 9.1 because of the adjustment made to $\sigma_{\bar{x}}$. In the first instance $\sigma_{\bar{x}} = 0.937$, and in this instance $\sigma_{\bar{x}} = 0.8492$.

Notice in Example 9.2 that the correction factor has *reduced* the standard error of the mean, ie reduced the variability of the sample means. This makes sense in that the larger the sample, the closer the sample mean will be to the population mean.

9.3   *Estimation*

In geriatric institutions, showering and dressing patients is very demanding on the time of staff. In order to plan for staffing a morning roster, a survey was taken to estimate how long, on average, this procedure takes. The showering and dressing of a sample of 15 patients were monitored. The times (in minutes) are listed below.

27 36 43 19 31 23 30 21 30 33 43 18 29 34 33

The mean time for the sample data (30 minutes) could be used as an estimate, but what was preferred was an estimate that covered a range of values. Not all patients would take 30 minutes to shower and dress, but it was felt that the job would take between 25 and 35 minutes, on average.

The above case is an example of estimation where both a *point estimate* ($\bar{x} = 30$ min.) as well as an *interval estimate* (25 – 35 min.) were considered. The idea of using sample statistics to estimate something of interest can be applied to estimating population parameters. For example, a sample mean $\bar{x}$ can be used to estimate the population mean μ, and the sample standard deviation s is used to estimate the population standard deviation σ. Such estimates are called point estimates because they provide a single-valued estimate of a parameter.

Sample statistics, however, are variable, and have a distribution with their own mean and standard deviation (the standard error). Therefore, point estimates may be somewhat misleading because of sampling variability. To get around this problem it is preferable to give an interval estimate which includes a range of possible values within which the population parameter is thought to lie.

In practice we usually do not know the true value of the population mean, μ, so we cannot say whether a particular sample mean is less than or greater than the population mean. So we establish a bracket or interval of values within which we think the true value of the mean might lie, keeping in mind the maximum error we are willing to accept.

Confidence intervals

We know from the Central Limit Theorem that sample means tend to be normally distributed, particularly for samples of 30 or more. We can use our knowledge of the normal distribution to find the endpoints of intervals, centred on the sample mean, which may contain the true population mean. These intervals are referred to as *confidence intervals*, as it is usual to specify a probability value associated with each interval, in much the same way as in Example 9.1(c). They are computed using the formula

$$\bar{x} \pm z.\sigma_{\bar{x}}$$

The wider the interval, the more probable that the interval contains the true population mean. The level of confidence placed on the interval determines the value of z to be used. Usual levels of confidence include 90%, 95%, and 99%. For 90% confidence intervals we require the values within which 90% of the distribution of sample means lie, so the area under the curve between the endpoints of the confidence interval will be 0.9000. To find the corresponding z-value we look up *half* this area in the z-tables. An area of 0.4500 gives a corresponding z-value of 1.645 (interpolating between 1.64 and 1.65). As the normal curve is symmetrical we have $z = \pm 1.645$.

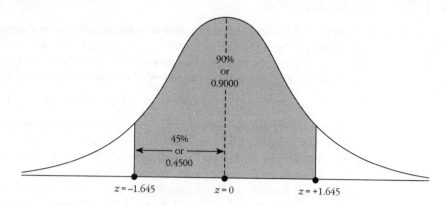

Figure 9.3 Normal curve showing a 90% confidence interval.

Using this method for the levels of confidence mentioned above, we obtain the following values for z:

Level of confidence	Corresponding z-value
90%	±1.645
95%	±1.96
99%	±2.575

Practical statistics for the health sciences

As these levels of confidence are nearly always used, the z-values are worth learning simply to save looking up the tables each time. Alternatively, reasonable approximations for z can be made using the values ±1.50, ±2.0, and ±2.50.

EXAMPLE 9.3

The times taken to shower and dress each of 15 geriatric patients were monitored and the following results (in minutes) were obtained. Assuming the distribution of times to be normal, and from previous large studies it is known that $\sigma = 7.625$, find a 95% confidence interval for the true average amount of time spent by staff in performing this task.

$$27 \quad 36 \quad 43 \quad 19 \quad 31 \quad 23 \quad 30 \quad 21 \quad 30 \quad 33 \quad 43 \quad 18 \quad 29 \quad 34 \quad 33$$

Solution

From the above information we have

$$\bar{x} = 30, \ \sigma = 7.625, \ n = 15, \ \sigma_{\bar{x}} = \frac{7.625}{\sqrt{15}} = 1.969$$

95% confidence gives $z = \pm 1.96$, so the interval for μ is given by

$$\bar{x} \pm z.s_{\bar{x}} = 30 \pm 1.96(1.969) = 30 \pm 3.859 = 26.14 \text{ to } 33.86$$

Confidence intervals using Minitab

To obtain confidence intervals using Minitab, the raw data needs to be available. The command ZINT will calculate a confidence interval based upon z-scores. The printout in Figure 9.4 demonstrates a 95% confidence interval for the sample of 15 patients mentioned in the worked example above. Note that in addition to specifying the level of confidence the ZINT command also requires a value for the standard deviation. The commands have been highlighted in bold type and the 95% confidence interval calculated by Minitab has been underlined.

```
MTB > print c1

Minutes
   27   36   43   19   31   23   30   21   30   33   43   18   29
   34   33

MTB > describe c1

                  N      MEAN    MEDIAN    TRMEAN    STDEV    SEMEAN
Minutes          15     30.00     30.00     29.92     7.63      1.97


                MIN       MAX        Q1        Q3
Minutes       18.00     43.00     23.00     34.00

MTB > zint 95 7.63 c1

THE ASSUMED SIGMA =7.63
```

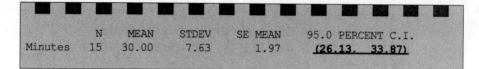

	N	MEAN	STDEV	SE MEAN	95.0 PERCENT C.I.
Minutes	15	30.00	7.63	1.97	(26.13, 33.87)

Figure 9.4 Minitab printout of 95% confidence interval for Example 9.3.

Increasing the degree of confidence required has the obvious effect of widening the interval, but increasing the sample size reduces the width of the confidence interval. The amount of spread in the population also has an effect upon the width of confidence intervals. The greater the spread, the wider the interval.

9.4 Estimation error

The error in an interval estimate refers to the deviation (difference) between the sample mean and the actual population mean. As we usually do not know the true value of the population mean, we can never be certain of the magnitude of the error of our estimate. We can, however, express a degree of certainty about the error in terms of a probability value. Since the confidence interval is centred on the sample mean, the maximum error can be no more than half the interval width, with the same probability as that associated with the confidence interval. So for a 95% confidence interval we can be 95% confident that the error will not exceed half the interval width.

We usually denote the maximum error associated with a confidence interval as e and by considering the formula used for finding a confidence interval we can define e. The confidence interval was defined earlier as $\bar{x} \pm z.\sigma_{\bar{x}}$. Diagrammatically this can be shown as follows:

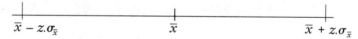

The distance from the centre of the interval to either endpoint represents the maximum size of the error associated with this particular interval. This distance is given by the value $z.\sigma_{\bar{x}}$. Therefore we have the following expression for the amount of error:

$$e = z.\sigma_{\bar{x}}, \text{ or } e = z\frac{\sigma}{\sqrt{n}}$$

The Minitab example above for the times taken to shower and dress geriatric patients gave a 95% confidence interval of 26.13 to 33.87 minutes. The width of this interval is simply the difference between the two values (33.87 − 26.13 = 7.74). The maximum error e then is half of this amount (3.87). Therefore we are 95% confident that the sample mean $\bar{x}$ differs from the true mean μ by an amount less than 3.87 minutes.

Practical statistics for the health sciences

9.5   *Estimating sample size*

Larger samples will give more accurate estimates of population parameters and therefore provide greater confidence in any interval estimates calculated. However, financial costs and time commitments very often limit the size of the sample. The *desirable* sample size may not be an *affordable* sample size. The question of concern is, 'What size sample do we need?' In particular, we often want to know the size of a sample such that the error in estimating the mean μ will be less than some specified amount e. In other words, we know what level of confidence we desire (z), we stipulate the amount of error we are prepared to tolerate (e) and we have some indication of the spread of the data to be collected (σ). From the equation for calculating the error we need to solve for n. This can be quickly determined by rearranging the formula used for describing the amount of error.

$$e = z\frac{\sigma}{\sqrt{n}} \Rightarrow n = \left(\frac{z.\sigma}{e}\right)^2$$

Hence, the necessary sample size will depend on any one, or some combination of, the following three quantities:

(a) the degree of confidence desired (z),

(b) the amount of dispersion among individual values in the population (σ),

(c) some specified amount of tolerable error (e).

EXAMPLE   **9.4**

In an effort to improve appointment scheduling, a doctor agreed to estimate the average time spent with each patient. A random sample of 49 patients yielded a mean of 30 minutes with a standard deviation of 7 minutes.
(a) Construct a 95% confidence interval for the true mean.
(b) What is the maximum probable error associated with the estimate in part (a)?
(c) What sample size would be necessary if the maximum error was to be no more than 1.5 minutes, assuming 95% confidence?

Solution
We have the following summary from the information given:

$$\bar{x} = 30,\ s = 7,\ n = 49,\ s_{\bar{x}} = 1,\ z = 1.96$$

(a)   The 95% confidence interval for $\mu = \bar{x} \pm z.s_{\bar{x}} = 30 \pm 1.96(1) = 30 \pm 1.96$

Therefore the 95% interval for μ is 28.04 to 31.96.

(b)   The maximum probable error is $e = z.s_{\bar{x}} = 1.96$ minutes.

(c)   To find the required sample size n given that $e = 1.5$, we have

$$n = \left(\frac{zs}{e}\right)^2 = \left(\frac{1.96(7)}{1.5}\right)^2 = 83.66.\ \text{Therefore choose a sample of size 84.}$$

In Example 9.4 the population standard deviation (σ) is unknown, but since the sample size is greater than 30 the sample standard deviation (s) can be used as a good approximation for σ, and the same formulae apply.

9.6 Dealing with small samples

We know from the Central Limit Theorem that the distribution of sample means is normal provided that the samples are large, ie $n \geq 30$, or the population is normal. For large sample sizes the sample standard deviation s is a good approximation for σ, but for $n < 30$ this is not so. To compensate for this we make use of the *t*-distribution, rather than the *z*-distribution used in previous examples. The *t*-distribution is similar to the *z*-distribution except that it is slightly *fatter* in the tails and not quite as *humped* towards the centre. It is also different in that for each particular sample size there is a slightly different *t*-distribution. This is shown in Figure 9.5, where several *t*-distributions are compared to the usual *z*-distribution. Notice that as the size of the sample increases the *t*-distribution gets closer to the *z*-distribution.

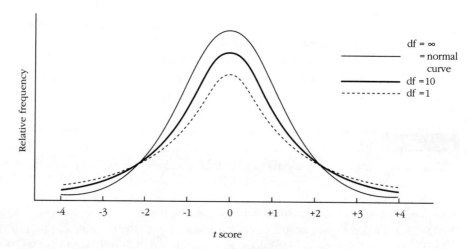

Figure 9.5 Comparison of some *t*-distributions with the usual *z*-distribution.

Before using the *t*-distribution, particularly with a small sample, satisfy yourself that the population from which the sample was taken is approximately normal. If the population *is* approximately normal, values for this distribution may be calculated using the following formula:

$$t_{n-1} = \frac{\bar{x} - \mu}{s_{\bar{x}}}$$

The subscript $n-1$ refers to the *degrees of freedom* associated with this statistic, which relate to the *number* of values that are free to vary when calculating the statistic. Imagine 20 students waiting outside a room in which there are exactly 20 chairs available for them to sit on. If each student is permitted to enter the room one at a time then 19 of them will have a choice of more than one seat. The last student will have no choice at all.

This is a similar concept to degrees of freedom. The *t*-statistic, as we have seen above, makes use of the sample standard deviation s, which is defined in terms of the mean, so we need to know $\bar{x}$. When calculating the mean, all scores can vary. But if $\bar{x}$ is fixed, all of the scores are free to vary, except one; that is, $n-1$ of the scores are free to vary. This can easily be shown with a simple example. Think of five numbers that have an average equal to 10. The first four numbers can be any value you like, but because we know that the mean must equal 10, the value of the fifth number is fixed.

So there are $n-1$ degrees of freedom associated with s, and in calculating t we need to use s. Therefore there are $n-1$ degrees of freedom associated with t.

Tables for the t-distribution are usually slightly different than those for the z-distribution. The body of the t-tables contain t-values rather than probability values, which usually appear across the top row of the t-tables. The different values for the degrees of freedom appear down the left-hand side of the tables. To find the t-value associated with a 95% confidence interval and a sample of size 15, proceed as follows:

1   Determine the area in the tail (95% confidence implies 2.5% in each tail).

2   Determine the degrees of freedom (for $n = 15$, d.o.f. $= 14$).

3   Find the appropriate t-value ($t = \pm 2.1448$).

If a z-score were required we would use $z = \pm 1.96$, regardless of the sample size. A comparison with z will show that, for $n > 30$, t provides a good approximation to z.

EXAMPLE   **9.5**

A random sample of eight packets of a certain brand of breakfast cereal has an average fibre content of 3.6 g per 100 g and a standard deviation of 0.9 g per 100 g. Calculate a 99% confidence interval for the true average fibre content for this particular brand of breakfast cereal, assuming that the fibre content is normally distributed.

Solution
From the information given,

$$\bar{x} = 3.6, \; s = 0.9, \; n = 8, \; s_{\bar{x}} = \frac{0.9}{\sqrt{8}} = 0.3182$$

As $n < 30$ and σ is unknown, we use t.

With 99% confidence the appropriate tail area is 0.005.
For $n = 8$ we have 7 degrees of freedom.
The appropriate t-value is therefore $t_7 = 3.499$.
The required interval for μ is therefore given by

$$\bar{x} \pm t_{n-1} s_{\bar{x}} = 3.6 \pm 3.499(0.3182) = 2.487 \text{ to } 4.713$$

9.7   *Using Minitab to obtain t-intervals*

The command TINT (short for TINTERVAL) is used to obtain the required t-intervals in Minitab. When obtaining confidence intervals you may specify the desired level of confidence and must specify which column contains the data. If no confidence level is stated the default setting is for a 95% confidence level. Figure 9.6 shows a 95% t-interval for the sample of 15 times taken to shower and dress geriatric patients considered earlier. (Compare the width of this t-interval with that obtained using the z-interval.) Note also that Minitab automatically uses the standard deviation of the sample when calculating a t-interval. This means that the raw data needs to be accessible to Minitab.

```
MTB > tint c1

              N      MEAN    STDEV    SE MEAN     95.0 PERCENT C.I.
Minutes      15      30.00    7.63      1.97       (25.78,   34.22)
```

Figure 9.6 95% *t*-interval for the sample in Example 9.3.

Interval estimates based upon sample means will not always contain the population mean. A 95% confidence interval implies that 95% of similarly constructed intervals, based upon samples of the same size, can be expected to include the population mean. This means that 5% can be expected *not* to include the population mean. Of course we can never be really sure if our particular confidence interval is one of the 95% group that are right or one of the 5% group that are wrong. The narrower the confidence interval the better, and this can be achieved by increasing the sample size or reducing the degree of confidence, or by minimising the measurement error through greater precision.

CENTRAL LIMIT THEOREM

1 What is the distinction between statistics and parameters?

2 Which of the following statements concerning the Central Limit Theorem is correct?
   (a) The CLT states that the mean of the distribution of sample means is equal to μ.
   (b) The CLT states that for large samples the sample mean is always equal to μ.
   (c) The CLT states that for large samples the distribution of the sample mean is approximately normal.

3 When a random sample of size n is drawn from a normal population with mean μ and standard deviation σ, the sampling distribution of the sample mean will be:
   (a) exactly normal,
   (b) approximately normal,
   (c) binomial, or
   (d) none of the above.

4 Which of the following statements is/are always true, regardless of the sample size drawn?
   (a) The mean of the sampling distribution of the means is equal to the mean of the population from which the samples were drawn.
   (b) The standard error of the mean will be greater than the standard deviation of the population from which samples were drawn.
   (c) The standard error will increase as sample size increases.
   (d) The sampling distribution of the mean has precisely the same scatter as the parent population from which the samples were drawn.

5 The Central Limit Theorem states that the distribution of sample means will be approximately normal if the sample size is large. In what way does the sample size depend upon the nature of the population distribution for sample means to be approximately normal?

6 Suppose samples of size 4 are drawn from a normally distributed population. What can be said about the distribution of the means of these samples?

7 Find the mean and variance of the distribution of sample means for samples of size 100 taken from a normal distribution with a population mean of 100 and variance of 16.

8 Find the mean and standard deviation of the sample means for samples of size 64 taken from a continuous population with mean 50 and standard deviation 20.

9 Assume that the times measured by 3-minute egg-timers is normally distributed with $\mu = 3$ mins and $\sigma = 0.2$ mins. If we test samples of 25 timers, find
   (a) the proportion of egg-timers with times measuring less than 2.9 minutes,
   (b) the number of egg-timers measuring more than 3.05 minutes,
   (c) the probability of the sample mean being less than 2.96 minutes,
   (d) the time that would be exceeded by 95% of the sample means.

10 An auditor is going to sample 64 charge accounts from many thousands active at a large department store. If the average balance owed for all of the store's accounts is $75 and the standard deviation for all accounts is $100, what is the probability that the sample mean of the balances owed among the 64 accounts sampled by the auditor is below $70?

11 The weight of baggage checked by airline passengers is a random variable with a mean of 50 kg and a standard deviation of 15 kg. If 100 passengers board the plane, the legal baggage limit for a particular aircraft is 5250 kg. What is the probability of exceeding the baggage limit?

12 An advertising agency has determined that the average cost to develop a 30-second commercial is $20 000. The standard deviation is $3000. What are the chances of obtaining a sample mean of $20 300 or more, if a random sample of 50 commercials is selected?

13 Suppose the advertising agency in Question 12 wishes to establish a pricing policy for their 30-second commercials, assuming a mean cost of $20 000 and a standard deviation of $3000.

(a) What are the chances of any given commercial costing between $19 500 and $22 000?

(b) What is the probability of a sample of 36 commercials having an average cost between $19 500 and $22 000?

(c) Explain why these probabilities are different.

14 From a normal distribution with a mean of 250 and a standard deviation of 20, how large a sample must be taken if the probability that the sample mean falls between 240 and 260 is 0.95?

15 The standard error of the mean for random samples of size 36 is 2. How large must the size of the sample be if the standard error is to be reduced to 1.2?

CONFIDENCE INTERVALS

16 What is the difference between a point estimate and an interval estimate for a parameter?

17 What is meant by the term *error*?

18 As the sample size n increases, all other things being equal, the width of a confidence interval for a population mean tends to:

(a) increase,

(b) decrease,

(c) stay the same, or

(d) increase sometimes and decrease sometimes depending on the value of the population mean.

19 If a researcher constructs 95% confidence intervals, then which of the following statements is true?

(a) 95% of the time the computed interval will include the sample mean.

(b) 5% of the time such intervals will not include the population value.

(c) In the long run, 95% of all sample means will fall within the interval.

(d) 95% of the time the interval will not include the population value.

20 The tax office is interested in estimating the tips earned by blackjack dealers in the growing number of casinos around Australia. To arrive at an estimate, a sample of 40 dealers was selected on a randomly selected day. The average amount received in tips for the sample was $55.80 with a standard deviation of $9.30.

(a) Estimate the true average amount earned in tips by all blackjack dealers using a 95% confidence interval.

(b) Find a 90% confidence interval.

21 Each January a polling company conducts a survey of television viewers in an attempt to estimate the average number of hours spent by Australians watching television per day. A recent report showed that for a random sample of 1700 the mean time spent watching television was 7.2 hours with a standard deviation of 2.3 hours.

(a) What is the point estimate for the average number of hours spent by Australians watching TV per day?

(b) Calculate a 95% confidence interval for the true average number of hours Australians spend watching TV.

22 Nurses at a blood bank take 600 mL from each donor on average. Doubts have been expressed regarding the accuracy of the collection. A sample of 10 blood packs are randomly selected and carefully measured. The results showed a mean of 593 mL with a standard deviation of 13 mL.

(a) Construct a 95% confidence level interval for the true volume of blood.

(b) Does the interval estimate obtained support the statement that each blood pack will contain 600 mL?

(c) How likely is it that on average the nurses *do* take 600 mL from each donor?

23 A local television station has added a consumer spot to its nightly news. The consumer reporter has recently bought 10 bottles of aspirin from a local chemist and has counted the aspirins in each bottle. Although the bottles advertised 500 aspirins, the reporter found the following numbers:

491, 487, 496, 504, 483,
490, 497, 507, 481, 495

The reporter claimed that this was an obvious case of the public being cheated. Comment. (Hint: Find a 95% confidence interval for the average number of aspirins based upon the sample data above.)

24 The following confidence intervals estimate the mean age of patients suffering from sexually transmitted diseases in a particular city, and have been constructed from three different simple random samples. Assume the distributions of age to be normal.

Sample	Lower limit	Upper limit
a	19.0	30.0
b	20.0	31.9
c	22.0	30.0

If the three samples used the same estimate for the standard deviation of the ages, and all three intervals were constructed using 95% confidence, which sample was the largest? Explain how you know this. Which sample was the smallest? How do you know this?

25 Referring to Question 24, suppose sample b was of size 36 and the standard deviation was 16. Approximately what level of confidence should be associated with this interval?

26 Referring to Question 24, suppose each of the three samples contained 60 observations, and all three intervals were constructed using 80% confidence. Which sample had the smallest standard deviation? Explain.

27 Compute the standard error for each sample in Questions 24 and 26. Then determine what change in sample size would be needed to cut the standard error by one half.

ESTIMATION
28 A firm is converting machines it leases to updated versions. Forty machines have been converted so far. The average conversion time was 24 hours and the standard deviation 3 hours.
(a) Determine a 98% confidence interval for the average conversion time.
(b) What is the maximum probable error associated with the interval in part (a)?
(c) Determine an upper limit below which you can be 98% confident the true mean will lie.

29 A local group of pharmacists wished to estimate the mean expenditure per customer per month on prescription items. From a random sample of 100 customers it was found that the mean expenditure per customer was $47.50 with a standard deviation of $8.30.
(a) Construct a 95% confidence interval estimate for the true mean expenditure per customer.
(b) Suppose that instead of a sample of size 100 the pharmacists sampled only 20 customers. If the sample statistics remained the same, calculate the 95% confidence interval for this new sample size. What extra assumption would be required?
(c) What size sample would need to have been taken for the estimate of the mean to be within $1 of the true mean expenditure per customer?

30 A geriatric centre's personnel director was asked to investigate absenteeism among staff at their main centre. A random sample of 25 staff yielded a sample mean of 9.7 days absent in a year, with $s = 4.0$ days. Calculate 95% confidence interval estimates for:
(a) the average number of days absent per member of staff.
(b) the average number of days absent for the staff given that 150 are employed in total.
If the personnel director also wishes to take a survey from one of the hostels associated with the centre:
(c) What sample size is needed if he wishes to be 95% confident of being correct to within ±1.5 days, assuming that $\sigma = 4.5$?
(d) What sample size is needed if he wishes to be 99% confident of being correct to within ±1.2 days, assuming that $\sigma = 4.5$?

31 Determine the sample size needed to estimate the mean waiting time at an outpatient clinic if the maximum error is to be 5 minutes using a 90% confidence level. Waiting time is known to be normally distributed with a standard deviation of 12 minutes.

REVISION

32 How large a sample would be required in order to estimate with 98% confidence the mean slack time per employee (in hours) with a maximum error of ±1 hour? Assume that the distribution of slack time per employee is normal with a standard deviation of 4 hours.

33 A survey is planned to determine the average annual family medical expenses for employees of a large company. The company wishes to estimate this average to within ±$50 of the true value. A pilot study has indicated that the standard deviation of family expenses is $400.

(a) What size sample would be necessary to obtain the desired accuracy with 92% confidence?

(b) What accuracy would be achieved with 98% confidence using a sample of 64 employees?

34 For samples of $n = 400$ from a normal distribution with $\mu = 24$ and $\sigma = 6$, find the mean and standard deviation of the distribution of sample means.

35 A bicycle shop sells 10-speed bicycles and offers a maintenance program to its customers. The manager has found the average repair bill during the maintenance program's first year to be $15.30 with a standard deviation of $7.00.

(a) What is the probability that a random sample of 40 customers will have a mean repair cost exceeding $16.00?

(b) What is the probability that the mean repair cost for a sample of 100 customers will be between $15.10 and $15.80?

36 The University Sports Club is in the process of establishing a policy on how long a tennis court may be reserved at any one time. To help make this decision, the club managers selected a random sample of 25 tennis matches and determined the mean time for completion to be 75 minutes. What is the probability of finding a sample mean less than or equal to this, if the true average completion time is 90 minutes with a standard deviation of 20 minutes?

37 A study of the health records of a large group of deceased males who smoked at least one pack of cigarettes daily over a 5-year period was conducted to determine the mean life span of all such individuals. A random sample of 16 health records for deceased smokers indicated an average life span of 65.7 years and a standard deviation of 3.4 years. Using these statistics, construct a 99% confidence interval for the true average life span μ for the population of male smokers who smoke at least one pack of cigarettes daily over a 5-year period. What assumptions have you made?

38 A health-care organisation conducted a study to estimate the average number of days that surgical patients are hospitalised. A random sample of 150 surgical patients yielded an average stay of 4.8 days and a standard deviation of 2.6 days. Find a 90% confidence interval for the mean number of days a surgical patient remains in hospital.

CHAPTER OUTLINE

10.1 Hypothesis testing
The concept of hypothesis testing and its applications.

10.2 Stating the hypotheses
Wording null and alternative hypotheses as logical counterparts.
Choosing at this stage, between a z-test and a t-test, then
deciding whether to accept or reject the null hypothesis.
Summary of the hypothesis testing procedure.

10.3 One-tailed versus two-tailed tests
Directional or non-directional alternative hypothesis, and the
consequences of this for the testing procedure and the
probability of rejecting the null hypothesis.

10.4 Type I and Type II errors
Making decisions based on probabilities. Possible errors and
their consequences.

10.5 Testing hypotheses using Minitab
Use and interpretation of the output of the ZTEST and TTEST
commands.

10.6 Estimating population proportions
Estimating population proportions and its applications.
Constructing confidence intervals for estimates of the
population proportion based on sample information. Limiting
the size of the error involved and the implications of this for
sample size.

10.7 Hypothesis tests for proportions
Applying the principles used for testing hypotheses about
population means to proportions.

CHAPTER TEN

Statistical inference

After reading this chapter you should be able to:
- express a research question in terms of null and alternative hypotheses;
- establish a statistical basis for accepting or rejecting the null hypothesis;
- decide whether a z or t-test statistic is appropriate for testing $\bar{x}$ vs μ;
- outline the steps to be taken to complete a hypothesis test;
- describe Type I and Type II errors in the context of a problem;
- use Minitab to perform hypothesis tests in situations where the appropriate test statistic is either a z or t statistic;
- interpret the p-value stated in Minitab output;
- use sample information to make estimates about population proportions;
- calculate confidence intervals for population proportions;
- calculate the possible error in the estimate of a population proportion;
- calculate the sample size needed to restrict the error of the estimate.

10.1 Hypothesis testing

A scientific approach to research begins when a researcher has an idea or a belief which they wish to test. This idea may have developed as a result of empirical observation or from reading previous research in the area. When the idea is formulated or worded in such a way that it can be tested, it becomes a hypothesis. Here are some examples:

- fluoride reduces the incidence of tooth decay;
- early discharge, post-delivery, has no adverse effects on mother or baby;
- smoking parents produce smoking children;
- smoking mothers deliver babies of low birth weights.

Since it is not possible to test such claims on a whole population, data must be collected from a sample and appropriate statistical tests applied. This chapter considers some of the tests we use to evaluate hypotheses such as those above.

In order to evaluate the *reasonableness* of a particular assumption, claim or belief, we do so in the light of what we observe. This is sometimes referred to as *empirical observation*. Sample statistics from our observations are used as the basis for determining whether or not a particular claim is reasonable. If the empirical results are too different from the hypothesis (ie what is being claimed) then the hypothesis is rejected. For example, a bus company claims that the average time for the 8.10 am bus to travel from the centre of town to the university is 15 minutes. This means that students who have to catch this bus will be on time for their 8.30 am lecture. A particular student who regularly travels on this bus makes *random* observations of the times taken for the trip over a 6-month period. Suppose that 50 observations were taken, and the average time was 18 minutes. What can be concluded from the observations with regard to the claim made by the bus company? Is the observed time difference just a chance difference, or is it an indication that the trip does take more than 15 minutes? In other words, *Does the observation differ significantly from what has been claimed?*

If random sampling is used to collect the empirical data, any sample statistics we might use will tend to vary naturally according to chance, or they will vary because something else is causing them to vary. By considering only chance variations we can make use of the methods developed in Chapter 9 based upon the Central Limit Theorem to investigate sample means. We know that it is highly unlikely, for example, for a sample mean to lie more than 2.5 standard errors from the true mean.

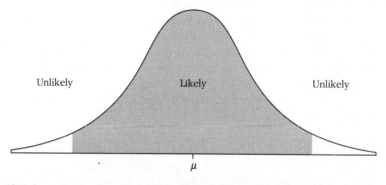

Figure 10.1 A sample mean is unlikely to lie more than 2.5 standard errors from the true mean.

For a sample mean to support a particular hypothesis it must lie in an area considered *likely* (or *acceptable*); if the hypothesis is true, we would expect this anyway. The distribution of the test statistic is used as the theoretical basis for determining what is acceptable and what is not acceptable. The points defining these regions are known as the *critical values* for the hypothesis test.

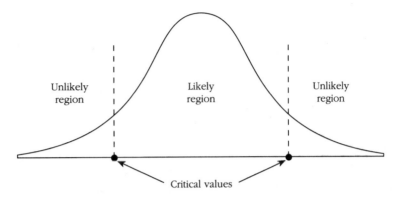

Figure 10.2 Critical points define the limits of the likely and unlikely areas.

The positions of the critical values are determined by stating the probability (risk) of making an incorrect decision by rejecting the null hypothesis (described in Section 10.2) when in fact it is true. These probabilities describe the area in the tail of the distribution, and are determined by the person conducting the test. Commonly used values are 10%, 5%, 2.5% and 1%. Stipulating such a percentage value defines the *level of significance* for the hypothesis test, which is often referred to as the *alpha level* (α-level) of the test. The α-level or the level of significance for a test is the probability of rejecting the null hypothesis when it is true.

One might argue, for example, that if the bus company's claim of 15 minutes falls inside a 95% confidence interval based upon the sample mean of 18 minutes, then their claim can be considered to be reasonable. To use this approach we would need to assume that the travel times are approximately normally distributed and we would need to know the standard deviation for the travel times; both can be estimated from the sample data.

So hypothesis testing involves the use of information derived from random sampling to evaluate a claim about a population. We take the results from our observations or experiments and consider the probability of obtaining such results assuming that chance alone is responsible for any observed differences between what we find and what we believe to be the case. For hypothesis tests about the mean, the Central Limit Theorem provides us with a model that enables us to determine what is or is not acceptable.

10.2 Stating the hypotheses

We always formulate the problem in terms of two hypotheses. The first of these generally states that there is *no difference* between what is claimed and what is observed. This hypothesis is called the *null hypothesis*, and is denoted H_0. The second hypothesis presents the other options, which may be *more* or *less* than what is claimed, or simply *different* to H_0. This *alternative hypothesis* is denoted H_1. The usual procedure is to test whether H_0 is supported by the observed data, and to conclude by accepting or rejecting it in favour of H_1.

For the bus travelling time example in Section 10.1, we might have the following statements:

H_0:   the average travel time is 15 minutes, as claimed ($\mu = 15$).

H_1:   the average travel time is not 15 minutes ($\mu \neq 15$).

The alternative hypothesis may be expressed in a more specific manner by including a sense of direction in the statement. We would be more concerned if the average travel time was *more* than what was being claimed, so the alternative hypothesis could have been expressed with this in mind. That is,

H_0:   the average travel time is 15 minutes, as claimed ($\mu = 15$).

H_1:   the average travel time is more than 15 minutes ($\mu > 15$).

Rejecting a null hypothesis

By rejecting a null hypothesis H_0 we are saying that it is *unlikely* to be true given the nature of what we have observed or the data we have collected. Hence, we conclude that H_0 is false on the grounds that our observations do not reasonably match the claim of the null hypothesis. If H_0 seems to be reasonable in the light of our observations then we accept it, which means that we do not have sufficient reason not to believe it.

In many situations H_0 claims that a population parameter is equal to a particular value. The Central Limit Theorem states that the distribution of the sample means is likely to be normal, and it is more likely for any one sample mean to lie near the centre of the sampling distribution (ie the true population mean). If the null hypothesis claims that the true population mean is some particular value, then sample means lying close to the claimed value will tend to support H_0 while if they are far from the claimed value then H_0 may well be false.

In order to make the judgement about whether to accept or reject a claim, we establish critical values from the sampling distribution that will define areas that are *too far* from the centre of the distribution. If the sample statistic falls beyond these critical values, H_0 is rejected. For example, if a sample mean lies *two or more* standard errors from the hypothesised mean, we may decide to reject the null hypothesis, since the normal distribution tells us that less than 5% of sample means will lie two or more standard errors from the true population mean. A sample mean so far from the hypothesised value is not likely to occur as a result of chance alone.

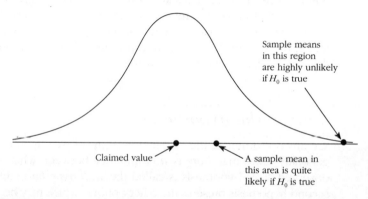

Sample means
in this region
are highly unlikely
if H_0 is true

Claimed value

A sample mean in
this area is quite
likely if H_0 is true

Figure 10.3 A normal curve with a claimed value (defining H_0), a close value supporting H_0 and a far value supporting H_1.

Practical statistics for the health sciences

The choice between *z* and *t*

In most practical situations σ is unknown, so theoretically we should use the *t*-distribution almost all the time (assuming that the underlying population is approximately normal). If the assumption of normality does not hold, we need to look at the size of the sample. For large samples, usually $n \geq 30$, the differences between *z* and *t*-values are small, so *z* can be used, mainly because of its convenience. (However, computer packages enable us to use the *t*-distribution beyond the tabled values.) For small samples from non-normal distributions other strategies are necessary; these are discussed in later chapters.

Procedure for hypothesis testing

The following summary presents an outline of the steps to follow when undertaking a hypothesis test. The example that follows uses the two concepts of confidence intervals and probability values to test the relevant hypothesis. Both techniques have been met previously in Chapter 9.

1   Clearly state both null and alternative *hypotheses*.

2   Decide which *test statistic* is appropriate, give reasons.

3   Determine the *rejection* region by choosing a suitable α-level.

4   Locate the *sample statistic* with respect to the rejection region — H_0 can only be rejected if the sample statistic lies within the rejection region.

5   State the *conclusion* (resulting from step 4) in the context of the problem.

EXAMPLE 10.1

A new drug has been released by a drug company to provide relief from the effects of hayfever. The drug company claims that each dose will provide total relief for an average of 12 hours. A group of doctors decides to test the drug company's claim by asking a random sample of 50 patients (known sufferers of hayfever) to keep a record of the hours of relief provided by this new drug. It was found that the average time relief was 11 hours, with a standard deviation of 1.5 hours. At a 5% level of significance, what can the doctors conclude?

Method A: The confidence interval approach
Solution
From the information above we have the following summary:

$$n = 50, \ \bar{x} = 11.5, \ s = 1.5, \ s_{\bar{x}} = \frac{1.5}{\sqrt{50}} = 0.2121, \ \alpha = 0.05$$

1   H_0:   The average relief is 12 hours; ie $\mu = 12$.

   H_1:   The average relief is not 12 hours; ie $\mu \neq 12$.

2   As *n* is large we can use the *z*-distribution.

3   For $\alpha = 0.05$, and a two-tailed test, the combined area in both tails of the distribution is equal to 0.05, therefore in one tail the area is only 0.025. The corresponding *z*-score is $z = \pm 1.96$. This value is obtained from the *z*-tables by looking for an area corresponding to 0.4750 in the body of the table.

A 95% confidence interval based upon the hypothesised mean is therefore:

$12 \pm 1.96(0.2121) = 12 \pm 0.4157 = 11.58$ to 12.42

So we will reject H_0 if the sample mean lies outside this interval.

4   The sample mean $\bar{x} = 11.5$ lies outside the confidence interval above, so we can reject the null hypothesis.

5   We conclude that the sample data does not support the drug company's claim at the 5% level of significance. It would appear that the period of relief *is not* 12 hours.

Method B: The probability value approach
Solution
From the information above,

$$n = 50, \ \bar{x} = 11.5, \ s = 1.5, \ s_{\bar{x}} = \frac{1.5}{\sqrt{50}} = 0.2121, \ \alpha = 0.05$$

1   H_0:   The average relief is 12 hours; ie $\mu = 12$.

    H_1:   The average relief is not 12 hours; ie. $\mu \neq 12$.

2   As n is large we can use the z-distribution.

3   For $\alpha = 0.05$ (ie combined area in both tails of the distribution is equal to 0.05) the area in each tail of the distribution is therefore 0.025. If H_0 is true we calculate the probability of obtaining a sample mean as extreme as 11.5. If this p-value is less than 0.025 we reject H_0.

4   For $\bar{x}$ we obtain $z = \dfrac{11.5 - 12}{0.2121} = -2.36$.

    Pr(beyond z) = 0.5000 − 0.4909 = 0.0091 = p-value < 0.025.

5   The obtained p-value is less than 0.025; therefore we reject H_0.

10.3   *One-tailed versus two-tailed tests*

Example 10.1 is an example of what we call a two-tailed hypothesis test. The wording of the alternative hypothesis, $\mu \neq 12$, implies that a significant variation in either direction will lead to a rejection of the null hypothesis. Two-tailed tests are used whenever variation in either direction is critical. For example, in pieces of material that are sewn together to make clothes, engine parts that fit together, or the amount of a drug in a tablet. In each of these instances, *excess* is just as critical as *insufficiency*. When dealing with two-tailed tests the α-level is spread equally between both ends of the sampling distribution.

One-tailed tests can either be *left-tail* tests or *right-tail* tests. Left-tail tests are useful when you are testing to see if minimum requirements have been met. For example, net weight, tensile strength or product life. Right-tail tests, on the other hand, are used when maximum standards must not be exceeded, such as in radiation exposure and exhaust emissions. In Example 10.1 it may have been appropriate to have used a left-tailed test, because average relief times greater than 12 hours strengthen the drug company's claim, in that longer relief is a favourable outcome for the company. If this were to be the case then the alternative hypothesis would be reworded as

    H_1:   The average relief time is *less* than 12 hours; ie $\mu < 12$.

In addition, $\alpha = 0.05$ implies that $z = -1.645$. This time the significance level refers to the area in the left tail (5%), which leaves 45% between the edge of the critical region and the centre of the sampling distribution. Hence the z-score given above. Notice that for one-tailed tests the edge of the critical region is slightly closer to the centre of the sampling distribution than for two-tailed tests, given the same level of significance. This makes it easier to reject a null hypothesis for a given α-level.

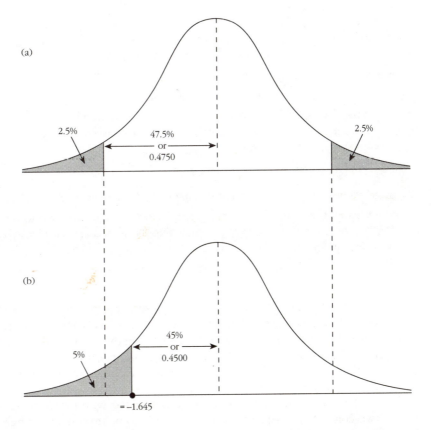

Figure 10.4 Critical areas for (a) two-tailed test with $\alpha = 0.05$, and (b) one-tailed test with $\alpha = 0.05$.

EXAMPLE **10.2**

A hospital spokesperson claimed that the average account for major surgery last year did not exceed $20,000. Auditors assigned to study these accounts select nine from a list of last year's total of 60 accounts provided by the hospital administration. They find the mean account to be $23,400. The sample standard deviation was found to be $6,000. What can the auditors conclude if they decide to use a 5% level of significance and it is known that the distribution of such accounts is normal?

Solution
 Note: We will use t because $n < 30$ and σ is unknown. We also need to use the *finite correction factor* because nine accounts were chosen out of 60, which is 15%; ie $n > 5\%$ of N. So

EXAMPLE 10.2 cont.

$$n = 9, \; N = 60, \; \bar{x} = 23400, \; s = 6000, \; \sqrt{\dfrac{N-n}{N}} = 0.922$$

$$\text{so adjusted } s_{\bar{x}} = \dfrac{6000}{\sqrt{9}} \, (0.922) = 1844$$

We will use the confidence interval approach because probability values are inconvenient when using the t-distribution.

1 H_0: states that the mean does not exceed $20,000; ie $\mu \leq 20000$.

   H_1: states that the mean is significantly greater; ie. $\mu > 20000$.

2 As $n < 30$ and σ is unknown, we use the t-distribution.

3 For $\alpha = 0.05$ the corresponding t-score with eight degrees of freedom is given by $t_8 = +1.860$. Because we want a 5% one-tailed test, each tail has 5%, therefore we are actually calculating a 90% confidence interval, given by:

$$20000 \pm 1.86(1844) = 16570.16 \text{ to } 23429.84$$

4 The sample value of $23,400 lies within this interval, so we cannot reject the null hypothesis.

5 We conclude that the sample data does not provide enough evidence to reject the claim made by the hospital at the 5% level of significance. It would appear that average account for major surgery does not exceed $20,000.

While the sample data may show a statistically significant difference at a particular α-level, whether or not this difference really matters is another issue. For example, when *E. coli* levels are measured at beaches in the summer it may well be that one beach has a significantly lower reading than another. However, the statistical significance of the difference is not a practical one if both beaches have levels that are considered unsafe for swimming.

Too often, statistical significance is equated with practical significance. The two concepts are separate issues and ought to be treated accordingly. By rejecting the null hypothesis, all we are saying is that the difference between the observed mean and that hypothesised under H_0 is not likely to have been caused by chance variations.

10.4   Type I and Type II errors

While it is important that samples are randomly chosen if probability theory is to be used to establish the significance of the results obtained, it is possible that such a sample may not represent the full range of data. There is therefore a chance that inferences made about the population may be wrong. For example, if the decision rule relies upon 95% of the sampling distribution lying within certain limits, then it follows that 5% of the sampling distribution will lie outside those limits, which might cause rejection of the null hypothesis when it is true. This is known as a *Type I error*, and the probability of it occurring is given by the α-level of the test. For example, if the α-level is set at 1% (ie 0.01) then the sample mean must be so far from the hypothesised mean that there is only a 1% chance that a sample with a mean as extreme, or more extreme, than this could occur if the null hypothesis were true.

Alternatively, we could make the opposite error of accepting the null hypothesis when it is in fact false. This is called a *Type II error*, and the probability of its occurrence is denoted by the Greek letter β (beta). Type II errors are more difficult to determine than Type I errors. Ideally we wish to make a correct decision, or at least design an experiment and test so as to minimise both α and β. Simply choosing a low α-level may not result in an equally low β-value. In some cases a decrease in α leads to an increase in β. One way to decrease both simultaneously is to use a larger sample size, but this may not always be possible.

The null hypothesis usually supports the *status quo*, so rejection of the null hypothesis may lead to change and changes are seldom undertaken lightly. As a result, Type I errors are considered to be more serious than Type II errors, so it is common to have small α-levels and to tolerate the sometimes slightly higher probabilities of making Type II errors. For example, the question of a patient's sanity can be very controversial. A patient will not be certified unless there is almost irrefutable evidence (very low α-level) because certification involves loss of liberties, etc. Ideally a balance between the cost of committing a Type I versus a Type II error should be achieved. Table 10.1 shows the possible decisions that can be made.

Table 10.1 Possible decisions, errors and probabilities in hypothesis testing.

Decision	H_0 true	H_0 false
Accept H_0	correct decision (probability $1-\alpha$)	Type II error (probability β)
Reject H_0	Type I error (probability α)	correct decision (probability $1-\beta$)

10.5   Testing hypotheses using Minitab

Minitab can carry out hypothesis tests using either the z or t-distributions using the commands ZTEST and TTEST. To use either of these commands the raw data must be available, and the hypothesised value of the mean needs to be indicated. The ZTEST command also requires an estimate of the population standard deviation. One-tailed tests are possible through the use of the subcommand ALTERNATIVE $= \pm 1$. The command for the left-tailed t-test that was used in Example 10.2 is

TTEST 20000 C1;
ALTERNATIVE $= -1$.

EXAMPLE   10.3

A student worked part-time for a firm delivering medical supplies and prescriptions to various locations as required by doctors, hospitals, patients, etc. The student was not happy with the $3.50 he was given for each delivery. His comment to his employers was that 'Everyone else seems to get at least $5 per delivery!' To check this claim, a random sample was taken of other

EXAMPLE   **10.3**   **cont.**

employees also involved in the delivery of these supplies. Payments for each delivery were noted and the following results obtained:

$3.00, $4.00, $4.00, $6.00, $5.00, $7.00, $10.00, $5.00, $5.00, $5.00, $5.00

On the basis of the evidence collected, and assuming the payments are normally distributed, what conclusion can be reached?

Solution

Several ways of expressing the hypotheses are possible. We have chosen to test the claim that the mean delivery payment is at least $5 (ie $\geq$$5)

1   H_0: $\mu \geq 5.00$
    H_1: $\mu < 5.00$
    The data was entered into Minitab and the following printout resulted.

```
MTB > print c1
Pay$
   3    4    4    6    5    7   10    5    5    5    5
MTB > ttest mean = 5 c1;
SUBC> alternative = -1.
TEST OF MU = 5.000 VS MU L.T.  5.000
          N     MEAN    STDEV    SE MEAN      T     P VALUE
Pay$     11    5.364    1.859      0.560    0.65       0.73
```

2   The p-value from the printout (0.73) is to be compared to the α-level of the test. If this p-value is less than the α-level we can reject H_0. As no α-level was suggested, we choose whatever we like, so let α-level be 5% (ie $\alpha = 0.05$).

3   As the obtained p-value > α-level, we cannot reject H_0. Therefore the claim made by the student appears to be justified. It is reasonable to conclude that the average payment per delivery is at least $5.00.

Notice that the Minitab printout in Example 10.3 includes a value T. This value is the t-statistic obtained from the data using the formula $t = \dfrac{\bar{x} - \mu}{s_{\bar{x}}}$. The value for μ is the value claimed according to the null hypothesis, in this case $\mu = 5$. The t-value obtained in this way represents the number of standard errors the sample mean is above or below the hypothesised mean. It can be compared to a critical t-value from the tables, and if greater in magnitude then H_0 can be rejected. The same argument applies when the z-distribution is used.

10.6   *Estimating population proportions*

Estimations of population proportions are such a regular feature of our daily lives that most of us take them for granted. Each of the following extracts, for example, were taken from one edition of the *Age* newspaper of 8 November 1993.

Women rarely consider their own interests when making personal insurance arrangements despite research showing that they control the domestic insurance purse strings in more than 82% of cases.

... about 50% of full-time university students below the age of 25 are working.

... the latest Time Morgan poll, taken in October, showed that support for the coalition government increased one point to 49.5%.

... there are still 240 million women in Asia alone who have no form of birth control, although 90% of them want it, according to the latest UN population report.

In each case above a sample proportion has been used to estimate a population proportion that is of interest to the researcher. In keeping with the usual practice of using Greek letters to represent population parameters, we represent the population proportion by the Greek letter π (pi). The sample proportion is represented by the corresponding Roman letter, p.

The sample proportion is the ratio of the number of people in the sample possessing a certain characteristic of interest to the total number of people in the sample. That is,

$$p = \frac{\text{number of 'successes'}}{\text{total sample size}} = \frac{x}{n}$$

The estimation of population proportions is similar to the way we estimate population means. Sample proportions are approximately normally distributed provided that the samples are sufficiently large. Sufficiently large usually means that np and $n(1-p)$ should both be at least 5.

The distribution of sample proportions has a mean equal to the population proportion. This is usually written as $\mu_p = \pi$. The standard deviation of sample proportions is based on the binomial distribution and is defined as

$$\sigma_p = \sqrt{\frac{\pi(1-\pi)}{n}}$$

The values above can only be approximated in most real-life cases because we do not know the value of the population proportion π. However, by substituting the sample proportion p into the above equation, we get

$$\sigma_p \approx s_p = \sqrt{\frac{p(1-p)}{n}}$$

The quantity s_p is an estimate of σ_p, which is the standard error of the proportion.

Confidence intervals for proportions

Interval estimates for population proportions are found in much the same way as those for population means. A confidence interval for the population proportion π, based upon a sample proportion p, is given by

$$\text{C.I.} = p \pm z\sqrt{\frac{p(1-p)}{n}}$$

Where necessary the finite correction factor is used to adjust the standard error, s_p. In this case the finite correction factor can be included under the square root sign:

$$\text{C.I.} = p \pm z\sqrt{\frac{p(1-p)(N-n)}{nN}}$$

If by chance one of the confidence limits is either negative, or greater than one, common sense dictates that we replace it by 0 or 1. By definition π cannot be less than zero, or more than one.

EXAMPLE **10.4**

A recent survey of 1000 people showed that 40% were members of some kind of health benefits fund. Estimate the true proportion of people who are members of a health benefits fund with 95% confidence.

Solution
From the above information,

$$n = 1000, \; p = 0.40, \; s_p = \frac{0.40(1 - 0.40)}{1000} = 0.0155$$

For 95% confidence we have $z = \pm 1.96$, so the required interval for π is

$$p \pm z.s_p = 0.40 \pm 1.96(0.0155) - 0.40 \pm 0.0304$$

Therefore the 95% confidence interval for π is 0.37 to 0.43. That is, 370 to 430 people are members (with 95% confidence).

Error

The amount of error in an interval estimate is one-half of the width of the interval.

Therefore the equation $p \pm z \sqrt{\dfrac{p(1-p)}{n}}$ can be thought of as $p \pm e$, and the error with respect to estimating proportions is

$$e = z \sqrt{\frac{p(1-p)}{n}}$$

You can see that as the level of confidence increases (ie z increases) so too does the error, while larger samples result in smaller errors. However, the effect of the sample proportion is not so clear because as p increases $(1 - p)$ decreases. In fact when $p = 0.5$ the product $p(1 - p)$ will be $0.5(0.5) = 0.25$. No other value for p will yield a greater product than this, therefore the error will be greatest for $p = 0.5$.

Estimating sample size

One of the most frequent uses of the error formula is to determine the sample size necessary to achieve a required degree of precision. If we solve for n, we obtain

$$e = z \sqrt{\frac{p(1-p)}{n}}$$

which implies that

$$n = \frac{z^2 p(1-p)}{e^2}$$

If the sample has been drawn from a population of known size N, we can obtain a smaller estimate for n using the finite population correction factor. In this case we use:

$$n = \frac{z^2 \, p(1-p)}{e^2 + z^2 \, p(1-p)/N}$$

EXAMPLE 10.5

A recent survey of people living in Australian cities showed that 40% were members of some kind of health benefits fund. If 2500 were surveyed, find the estimation error using 95% confidence.

Solution
From the above information,

$$n = 2500, \ p = 0.40, \ s_p = \sqrt{\frac{0.40(1-0.40)}{2500}} = 0.0098$$

For 95% confidence we have $z = \pm 1.96$, so the estimation error is

$$e = z.s_p = 1.96(0.0098) = 0.0192$$

EXAMPLE 10.6

A local town council was interested in the viability of opening a health benefits fund office in their particular town of 1500 people. As a part of their submission they had to estimate the proportion of people in the town who would be prepared to make use of such a service. What size sample should they use to achieve a 95% confidence interval for the population proportion if the tolerable error was to be limited to 1.5%?

Solution
From the above information

$$N = 1500, \ e = 0.015, \ z = \pm 1.96, \ \text{use } p = 0.40$$

For this example we have chosen to use the proportion (40%) from the survey of Australian cities in Example 10.5. If this information had not been available we would have used $p = 0.50$.

(a) If we choose not to use the correction factor, we have

$$n = \frac{z^2 p(1-p)}{e^2} = \frac{3.8416 \times 0.4 \times 0.6}{0.000225} = 4098$$

This results in a sample size greater than the population of the town!

(b) By using the correction factor we can obtain a considerable saving:

$$n = \frac{N z^2 p(1-p)}{N e^2 + z^2 \, p(1-p)} = \frac{1500 \, (0.922)}{1500 \, (0.0002) + 0.922} = 1131.75$$

So use $n = 1132$

The council now has to decide whether or not it is worth their while to practically sample the entire town. It may be that the tolerable error could be relaxed. For example, if the error was relaxed to 2.5% the required sample size would be $n = 744$.

10.7   Hypothesis tests for proportions

When we test a hypothesis about a population proportion we are assuming that the value of π is not known for sure, but there will be some particular value of π under consideration. The null hypothesis assumes that the proportion has a specific value $\pi = \pi_0$. The subscript is used to remind us that we are using the value being claimed by the null hypothesis. The calculation of the standard error, σ_p is based upon this value. If we reject H_0 and obtain a confidence interval for π, then we must use s_p to estimate σ_p since we still do not know π.

When testing hypotheses concerning π we will use the same procedure discussed in the previous section when we were testing hypotheses concerning the population mean μ. But remember that the methods used in this section should only be used when the sample sizes are sufficiently large; that is, as long as np and $n(1 - p)$ are both ≥ 5.

EXAMPLE   10.7

A university spokesperson claims that the proportion of nursing students who fail to graduate within 4 years is at most 20%. A review committee obtained a random sample of 225 former nursing students and found that 162 had graduated within 4 years. Does this result lend support to the claim made by the university spokesperson? (Test at the 1% level of significance.)

Solution
From above we have the following summary

$$p = \frac{63}{225} = 0.28, \; \alpha = 0.01, \; \pi_0 = 0.20, \; \sigma_p = \sqrt{\frac{0.2 \times 0.8}{225}} = 0.0267$$

1    $H_0 : \pi \leq 0.20$ vs $H_1 : \pi > 0.20$

2   At $\alpha = 0.01$ and a one-tailed test, $z = +2.33$.

3   From the data we obtain $z = \dfrac{p - \pi}{\sigma_p} = \dfrac{0.28 - 0.20}{0.0267} = +2.996$

4   From the tables, the probability of $z \geq 2.996$ is about 0.0013. That is, the p-value for this test is $p = 0.0013$ which is less than $\alpha = 0.01$, so we can reject the null hypothesis and conclude that the spokesperson's claim is false. It seems that the proportion of nursing students who do not graduate within 4 years is higher than 20%. A 95% confidence interval for the proportion who do not graduate within 4 years is given by $p \pm z.s_p$. Hence we have:

$$p \pm z.s_p = 0.28 \pm 1.96 \sqrt{\frac{0.28 \times 0.72}{225}} = 0.28 \pm 0.0587$$

so that the 95% confidence interval for the population proportion is 0.22 to 0.34.

Instead of using the p-value as the basis of the hypothesis test, we could just as easily have used the value $z = 2.996$ obtained from the data in step 3. This value would be compared to the critical z-value of 2.33 which is obtained from the tables. In this case the obtained value is beyond 2.33, so we have enough evidence to reject the null hypothesis.

1 True or false?

(a) Numerical measures used to summarise data collected from a population are called statistics.

(b) If the p-value associated with a test is $p = 0.016$, then an $\sigma = 0.01$ level test will result in acceptance of H_1.

2 What factors determine the choice between conducting a one-tailed test or a two-tailed test in a particular analysis?

3 True or false? The critical region is the region in which our sample statistic must fall if we are to *reject* the null hypothesis.

4 Choose the correct conclusion for the following statement. One should interpret the z-value associated with the α-level

(a) as the value beyond which good things happen,

(b) as the limit to the number of standard errors an observed value can lie from the value specified in the null hypothesis,

(c) as a numerical representation of the probability of success in making the correct decision, or

(d) as the limit to the distance from the value specified in the null hypothesis that can be expected to occur by chance or sampling variation if H_0 is true.

5 Which of the following significance levels will lead to the most frequent rejection of the null hypothesis?

(a) .10,

(b) .001,

(c) .05, or

(d) .01.

6 Which of the following is correct regarding p-values?

(a) A p-value is the probability of obtaining the observed value of the test statistic or some value even more extreme if H_0 is true.

(b) A p-value is obtained from the probability distribution that correctly describes the sampling distribution of the test statistic when H_0 is true.

(c) A p-value allows a decision-maker to select different α-levels without having to obtain new critical values for the hypothesis test.

(d) All of the above.

(e) None of the above.

7 If the observed value of the test statistic falls in the acceptance region, should we

(a) accept the alternative hypothesis?

(b) accept the null hypothesis?

(c) not reject the null hypothesis, but not automatically accept it? or

(d) take another sample and evaluate it to see if the same results are obtained?

8 Use the information below to find the appropriate critical z-value, and determine the rejection region at the given level of significance.

(a) H_0: $\mu = 20$ vs H_1: $\mu \neq 20$; $\alpha = 0.05$

(b) H_0: $\mu \geq 30$ vs H_1: $\mu < 30$; $\alpha = 0.05$

9 A random sample of $n = 64$ observations from a population produced a sample mean of 81.2 and a standard deviation of 23.6. Suppose that you wish to show that the population mean μ is less than 85.

(a) Give the null hypothesis for the test.

(b) State the alternative hypothesis.

(c) What is the value of the test statistic?

(d) State the rejection region if $\alpha = 5\%$.

(e) What can you conclude from this?

10 It is claimed that a new treatment is more effective than the standard treatment for prolonging the life of terminal cancer patients. The standard treatment has been in use for a long time, and from records in medical journals the mean survival period is known to be 4.2 years. The new treatment is administered to 80 patients, and their duration of survival is recorded. The sample mean and the standard deviation are found to be 4.5 years and 1.1 years respectively. Is the claim supported by these results? Test at $\alpha = 0.05$. State the p-value.

11 A sample of 40 sales receipts from a university bookstore has a mean of $121 and a standard deviation of $10.20. Use these values to test H_0: $\mu = \$125$ vs H_1: $\mu < \$125$ at $\alpha = 0.05$.

12 A hospital's records show that the mean time to process a new admission is 18 minutes. Testing a new admission procedure, the hospital recorded the processing time for a random sample of 50 admissions. The results yielded a mean processing time of 16.9 minutes and a variance of 9.4 minutes. Is the new admission procedure significantly quicker than the existing admissions procedure? Use $\alpha = 0.01$.

13 A certain restaurant advertises that it puts a quarter of a pound (0.25 pounds) of beef in its burgers. A customer who frequents the restaurant thinks that the burgers contain less than 0.25 pounds of beef. With permission from the owner, the customer selects a random sample of 50 burgers and finds that the mean weight per burger is 0.23 pounds, with a standard deviation of 0.12 pounds. Test the restaurant's claim using a level of significance of 0.10.

14 The administrator of a large hospital is concerned about the number of days spent in the hospital by surgery patients. A random sample of 43 patients is chosen and the number of days spent in the hospital by each patient is recorded. Use this information (below) to determine if the average hospital stay for surgery patients significantly exceeds seven days. Use $\alpha = 0.05$.
10, 10, 4, 1, 4, 10, 10, 10, 8, 13, 7, 10, 11, 12, 15, 3, 5, 8, 6, 6, 8, 7, 8, 15, 11, 12, 11, 10, 9, 8, 5, 12, 5, 6, 8, 9, 12, 3, 4, 12, 7, 10, 7

15 In what situations should a t-test rather than a z-test be used?

16 For a one-sample t-test, how many degrees of freedom are associated with the following sample sizes?
(a) 24, (b) 10, (c) 19, (d) 4.

17 A random sample of eight cigarettes of a certain brand has an average nicotine content of 4.2 milligrams and a standard deviation of 1.4 milligrams. Is this in line with the manufacturer's claim that the average nicotine content does not exceed 3.5 milligrams? Use a 1% level of significance, and assume the distribution of nicotine content to be normal.

18 A car advertisement claims that with the new collapsible bumper system, the average body repair cost for the damages sustained in a collision impact of 40 km per hour does not exceed $800. To test the validity of this claim, 5 cars are crashed into a stone barrier at an impact force of 40 km per hour and their subsequent body repair costs are recorded. The mean and standard deviation are found to be $858 and $45 respectively. Does the data strongly contradict the claim made by the advertiser?

19 A pharmaceutical firm maintains that the average time for a drug to take effect is 24 minutes. In a sample of 19 trials the average time was 25 minutes, with a standard deviation of 2 minutes. Test the claim against the alternative that the average time is more than 24 minutes, with $\alpha = 0.01$.

20 As part of a larger study on the effect of sleep on student performance, a researcher is interested in finding whether students at college sleep significantly less than 8.0 hours per night on average. A random sample of 18 students are asked to record the approximate number of hours they sleep on a particular night. The results are summarised as follows:
$\Sigma x = 130.2$ $\quad \Sigma x^2 = 948.53$
What can the researcher conclude ?

21 In each case identify the null hypothesis (H_0) and the alternative hypothesis (H_1) using the appropriate symbol for the parameter of interest.
(a) A consumer group plans to test drive several cars of a new model in order to document that its average highway fuel consumption is less than 15 kilometres per litre.
(b) Subsoil water specimens will be analysed to determine if there is convincing evidence that the mean concentration of a chemical agent has exceeded 0.008.
(c) The setting of an automatic dispenser needs adjustment when the mean fill differs from the intended amount of 16 mL. Several fills will be accurately measured to decide if there is a need for resetting.

PROPORTIONS

22 A survey conducted by a health magazine concerned the issue of advertising by drug companies. Many respondents thought that companies that advertise have to charge more. Suppose a survey of 435 adults chosen at random from an Australian city finds 198 who agree with this viewpoint. Determine a 95% confidence interval for the proportion of all adults in the city who feel this way.

23 A sociologist interviews 120 out of the 650 families in an apartment complex and finds that 49 of them support the Landlord Rights Bill. Find a 90% confidence interval for the proportion of all families in the complex who support the legislation.

24 Many segments presented during news and current affairs broadcasts are preceded by a warning that some viewers may find some scenes offensive. After some particularly graphic footage of the effects of the famine in Somalia, a network conducted a survey to gauge viewer reaction to such scenes. A total of 863 people were interviewed. Of these, 244 saw the show and 27 of the 244 were offended by it. Determine 90% confidence intervals for:
   (a) the proportion of people who watched the show, and
   (b) the proportion of viewers who were offended.

25 What sample size should you take to estimate the population proportion to within ±0.05 with 95% confidence if:
   (a) a pilot study shows $p = 0.2$,
   (b) no pilot study results are available.
       (Hint: use $p = 0.5$.)

26 To obtain data for his thesis, a psychology major plans to interview people to determine whether their reaction to a certain situation is positive or negative. He wants to estimate the true proportion to within ±0.02 with a confidence level of 95%. If a pilot study shows 60 out of 100 people with positive reactions, how many should be interviewed?

27 The Gallup poll claims that 60% of people support the decision to increase state taxes made recently by the Government. An opposition poll decides to test this contention at the 0.05 level of confidence. What can be concluded if a random sample of 1460 people contains 835 who favour the proposition?

28 To test a hypothesis that, on average, at least 70% of consumers buying beer still prefer bottles to cans, a local brewery uses one day's sales to test the hypothesis at the 0.05 level. If the day's sales represent a random sample, what conclusions can be drawn if there are 1030 bottle sales and 520 can sales?

29 A particular company (Brand X) leads the soft drink market claiming 40% of all soft drink sales. To determine whether a certain town differs from this claim, a local bottler commissions a survey. The survey asks a total of 2137 people if they drink soft drinks, and if so what drink they prefer. Of 1203 people who drink soft drinks, 438 prefer Brand X. What level of significance is used if the conclusion is that the proportion in the town who prefer Brand X is not 0.40?

Progress review 4

1   A survey of mature-age students taken in 1992 showed that the average weekly amount spent on child care was $46.00. Assuming that the distribution of weekly expenditure on child care is normal, with $\sigma = \$15.60$, find the following:

   (a) The probability that a sample of size 36 will yield a sample mean less than $40.

   (b) The probability that a sample of size 36 will yield a sample mean between $40 and $50.

2   The speeds (in km/h) of 10 randomly selected vehicles travelling through a 45 km/h speed limit zone were taken, and the following results obtained:

   50.7, 49.6, 49.0, 49.1, 49.5, 48.3, 48.7, 49.7, 50.4, 48.1

   (a) What is a point estimate for the population mean μ?

   (b) Find a 90% confidence interval for μ.

   (c) What is the maximum error of estimate for μ?

3   A recent student assignment included the following Minitab printout showing a 95% confidence interval for the true average amount of time spent by students waiting for buses at a university campus. Using the printout below, answer the following questions.

```
MTB > tint 95 c1


               N      MEAN    STDEV    SE MEAN    95.0 PERCENT C.I.
Minutes   12    13.392    1.097     0.317    ( 12.694, 14.089)

MTB > nooutfile
```

   (a) Determine the sample mean.

   (b) What size sample was used for the survey?

4   A recent newspaper article stated that a random sample of size 144 from a certain population gave $\bar{x} = 150$ and $s = 36$. The article gave an interval estimate of the population mean μ as 150 ±4.95, but did not mention the level of confidence. What was the level of confidence used?

5   For the two claims below:

   (a) clearly state suitable null and alternative hypotheses,

   (b) give the type of critical region (right-tail, left-tail, or two-tailed), and

   (c) explain the meaning of a Type I error.

   Claim 1   The mean number of books borrowed per day from the college library is no more than 250.

   Claim 2   The mean number of families below the poverty line in a particular city is 2500.

6   A certain brand of cereal is packaged to contain 450 g, on the average. A consumer agency has received many complaints claiming that packages of the cereal contain less than 450 g. To test the claim that the mean content is at least 450 g the consumer agency randomly selects 100 packages and finds that $\bar{x} = 425$ with $s = 85$ g.

   (a) Complete the test at the 1% level of significance.

   (b) If the mean content really was 450 g how many times in 1000, on the average, would a sample mean result in a value of 425 g or less? (Use $\sigma = 85$ g.)

   (c) Based upon your answer in part (b), does the evidence appear substantial that the population mean μ is less than 450 g?

7   In the Minitab printout below are the results of a t-test on a sample of 15 data values. The values represent daily production of chocolate frogs (in kilograms) for 15 selected days using a new machine being tested by a company. (The company was interested in determining whether the new machine could produce in excess of 200 kg of chocolate frogs per day.)

```
MTB > ttest 200 c2;
SUBC> alt = 1.

TEST OF MU = 200.000 VS MU G.T. 200.000

             N      MEAN    STDEV    SE MEAN     T P VALUE
Frogwts     15    206.333   10.540     2.721   2.33  0.018

MTB > nooutfile
```

   (a) State the null and alternative hypotheses used in the test.
   (b) What can the company conclude?
   (c) What Minitab command would be used to obtain a 90% confidence interval for the data?

8   A survey of 4500 students conducted in 1992 highlights the impact the recession has had on students and their families. According to the survey, 34% of students received income from part-time work. Is this significantly less than the 41% of students who received income from part-time work in 1991? Test at the 5% level of significance.

9   To estimate the proportion π of passengers who had purchased tickets totalling more than $200 over a 12-month period, a railway official obtained a random sample of 200 passengers. It was found that 112 passengers had purchased tickets totalling more than $200 in the previous 12-month period.
   (a) What is a point estimate for π?
   (b) Find a 95% confidence interval for π.

11.1 Paired data

Experimental designs which result in paired data being collected. How each pair of scores may be directly compared, creating a single sample of difference scores.

11.2 Independent samples

Experimental designs which result in two independent sets of data being collected. The analysis of this data for both large and small samples using calculators and formulae, and using Minitab.

CHAPTER ELEVEN

Comparing means from two samples

After reading this chapter you should be able to:
- recognise experiments which will produce paired data and those which produce independent data;
- calculate difference scores for paired data and perform a one sample test on the difference scores;
- use Minitab to calculate difference scores and perform a one sample test;
- perform a z-test for two large independent samples;
- check the homogeneity of the variances of two small samples;
- decide whether a pooled variance should be calculated before performing a two-sample t-test for independent groups;
- perform a two-sample t-test for independent groups, by hand, if it is appropriate to calculate a pooled variance estimate; and
- use Minitab for two-sample t-tests, making appropriate use of the subcommands available.

Often we are faced with the need to compare scores from two groups of data. This occurs, for example, when teachers compare the performance of this year's students with that of last year's students, or when nurses compare a patient's present condition with that of yesterday or last week. These sorts of comparisons are usually made intuitively rather than on the basis of some sophisticated statistical analysis. The aim of this chapter is to introduce techniques that can be used when making comparisons between two sets of data.

In order to determine the correct procedure, three fundamental questions need to be answered:

1 Do the data sets consist of *paired observations*, or are the observations in each group *independent* of each other?

2 Have the data sets come from *normal distributions* or not?

3 Are the samples *large* or *small*?

A number of possibilities arise as a result of these questions, but in this chapter we will consider data that is normally distributed. How to deal with data which is not normal is discussed in Chapter 12.

11.1   Paired data

Data are considered to be *paired* when there is some *link* between subjects. Whether data are considered as paired or independent usually depends on the design of the experiment. If paired data are required, pairing is deliberately built into the experimental design. For example, a group of subjects may be tested under two conditions so that the first score of each subject may be directly compared with their second score. This is commonly used in *before-and-after* experiments, also called repeated measures design experiments, where the same subject is measured twice.

In other circumstances subjects may be chosen in such a way that pairs will undertake the same tests. Each pair is matched as closely as possible on all factors affecting the experiment except the control variable. These may include such factors as socio-economic status, educational background, race, attitudes and medical history. Studies on twins are examples of this style of experimental design.

When paired data are used we focus our attention on the *differences* between each pair of results. The more similar the data values the closer their average difference would be to zero. This is in fact what is stated by the null hypothesis: if the independent variable had the same effect under both circumstances then the mean of these difference scores should be close to zero.

The calculation of the differences between paired data values results in a single list of difference scores which can then be analysed using a single sample hypothesis test. These difference scores are also normally distributed. If the null hypothesis takes its usual form of assuming that there is no significant difference between the paired data values, the mean of the difference scores should be zero. This is stated as follows:

$$H_0 : \mu_D = 0$$

The alternative hypothesis may take any one of the following forms, depending upon the nature of the experiment:

$$H_1: \quad \mu_D \neq 0; \text{ or } \mu_D < 0; \text{ or } \mu_D > 0$$

Example 11.1 demonstrates the procedure to be followed for testing hypotheses involving paired data. The use of subscripts is included only to reinforce the fact that we are dealing with the differences between paired data values.

EXAMPLE 11.1

Seventeen severe headache sufferers undertook a short practical course in stress management techniques. Participants recorded the occurrence of headaches during the 4 weeks prior to the course and again during the 4 weeks immediately following the course. Can the claim that the stress management program results in a significant reduction in severe headaches be justified? Test at the 5% level.

Before	84	48	77	98	42	94	72	62	89	53	66	66	65	36	62	32	55
After	41	11	26	54	5	41	28	27	48	38	42	37	46	17	33	2	31
D	43	37	51	44	37	53	44	35	41	15	24	29	19	19	29	30	24

Solution

From the above data we have the following summary

$$n = 17; \quad \bar{x}_D = 33.76; \quad s_D = 11.39; \quad \frac{s_D}{\sqrt{n}} = 2.76$$

After checking that the data is normally distributed and noting that $n = 17$ we will use the t-distribution rather than z.

$H_0: \quad \mu_D = 0$. The program has not affected the number of headaches.
$H_1: \quad \mu_D > 0$. The program has decreased the number of headaches.

For $n = 17$ and with $\alpha = 0.05$ the critical t-score is $t_{16} = 1.746$

From the data we get: $t = \dfrac{\bar{x}_D - \mu_D}{s_D/\sqrt{n}} = \dfrac{33.76 - 0}{2.76} = 12.22$

As the obtained t-value (12.22) is beyond the critical value (1.746) we can reject H_0 and conclude that the stress management program significantly reduced the number of severe headaches.

Note: A decrease in the number of headaches produces a positive difference score when we take the after score from the before score; that is, we are subtracting smaller numbers from bigger numbers. This is why the alternative hypothesis was written the way it was. If the subtraction had been the other way around, most of the difference scores would have been negative and the alternative hypothesis would have reflected this by stating that $\mu_D < 0$.

We can use similar procedures to those in Example 11.1 to test for a specific increase or decrease. For example, we may wish to test the hypothesis that the stress management program will decrease the number of headaches by at least 20 per person. In this case we would have the following:

$$H_0: \quad \mu_D = 20 \quad \text{vs} \quad H_1: \quad \mu_D > 20$$

In this instance the test statistic would be calculated as follows:

$$t = \frac{\bar{x}_D - \mu_D}{s_D / \sqrt{n}} = \frac{33.76 - 20}{2.76} = 4.98$$

The alternative hypothesis here indicates a one-tail test, so with $\alpha = 0.05$ then the critical t-score is $t = \pm 1.746$. The value obtained is still beyond the critical value, so it would be reasonable to reject H_0 and conclude that, on average, the program reduced severe headaches by more than 20.

Note that when analysing the difference scores, negative difference scores need to be included as negative values, and zero scores are included as zeros (that is, they are not excluded).

Using Minitab for paired data

If the paired values are in C1 and C2 then the differences between each pair can be found by using the command LET c3 = c1 – c2.

To test the null hypothesis that the mean of these differences is zero against the alternative that the mean is greater than zero, use the command TTEST 0 c3 followed by the subcommand ALTERNATIVE = +1.

The following Minitab printout deals with the data from Example 11.1. The difference scores were obtained and put into C3 and then a *right-tail t-test* was carried out on the difference scores. A 95% confidence interval for the average difference score was obtained, and the hypothesis that the average difference score is greater than 20 was also tested. From the printout you can use the obtained t-values by comparing them with critical values from your t-tables. Alternatively, you may use the p-values from the printout by comparing them with the α-level. If the obtained p-value from the printout is less than the α-level then the null hypothesis can be rejected.

```
MTB > let c3 = c1 - c2
MTB > name c3 'Diff'
MTB > print c1 - c3

ROW    Before    After    Diff
  1        84        2      82
  2        10       11      -1
  3        77        6      71
  4        98       44      54
  5        42        5      37
  6        94       41      53
  7        12        2      10
  8        62       80     -18
  9        89       24      65
 10        43       38       5
 11        66       62       4
 12        66       57       9
 13        95       46      49
 14        36       17      19
 15        10       15      -5
```

Practical statistics for the health sciences

```
16    32    64    -32
17   105    55     50

MTB > ttest 0 c3;
SUBC> alternative = 1.

TEST OF MU = 0.000 VS MU G.T. 0.000

          N     MEAN    STDEV    SE MEAN      T   P VALUE
Diff     17    26.59    33.47       8.12   3.28    0.0024

MTB > tint 95 c3

          N     MEAN    STDEV    SE MEAN   95.0 PERCENT C.I.
Diff     17    26.59    33.47       8.12   (  9.38,   43.80)

MTB > ttest 20 c3

TEST OF MU = 20.000 VS MU N.E. 20.000

          N     MEAN    STDEV    SE MEAN      T   P VALUE
Diff     17    26.592   33.47       8.12   0.81    0.43
```

Figure 11.1 Minitab printout for data from Example 11.1.

The TTEST command uses $\alpha = 0.05$ as the default, so for a one-tailed test this means that the critical region consists of the whole 5% in one tail of the distribution. For a two-tailed test the 5% significance level is equally spread over both ends of the distribution. That is, the critical region consists of 2.5% at each end of the distribution. Changing the α-level has no effect on the Minitab command. In the example above, if a two-tailed test of the hypothesis that the average difference was 20 was required with $\alpha = 0.01$, then the correct Minitab command would remain the same (TTEST 20 c3). The obtained p-value of 0.43 would then be compared to $\alpha = 0.01$, or the obtained t-statistic of 0.81 could be compared to the critical value of t ($t = 2.921$) obtained from the tables. Either way, there is not enough evidence to reject the null hypothesis.

11.2   *Independent samples*

Imagine a situation where researchers want to determine whether or not there is a difference between two independent groups with regard to a particular variable. For example, they may wish to see if there is a significant difference between the examination scores of students who studied a particular course in 1988 and those of students currently studying the same course. Or industrial researchers may wish to see if there is a significant difference between the times taken by night-shift workers and day-shift workers to assemble certain components. Or a medical researcher may use blind drug trials, in which the experimental group takes a new drug and the control group takes a placebo.

In each of these cases we assume that the samples are *independent* if people have been chosen at random and in turn have been randomly allocated to either the control group or the experimental group. If we can also assume that the underlying populations are approximately normal, the procedures outlined in this section can be used to determine whether there is a significant difference between the means of samples taken from the respective populations. If the population means were actually equal, the difference between the two sample means would by implication be equal to or close to zero. It is this concept that forms the basis of the null hypothesis for testing the difference between two sample means. Now we need to consider a new distribution, the distribution of the *differences between two means*.

When we speak of the distribution of the difference between two sample means we need to consider all possible ways in which samples of size n can be taken from each population. We then need to consider all possible pairings of the samples from the two populations in order to obtain the distribution of the difference between the sample means.

For example, in a population of 100 people there are 75 287 520 ways of selecting a sample of size 5. If a second population consists of only 70 people then there are 12 103 014 different ways of selecting a sample of size 5. To get all possible pairings of the samples from the two populations, we multiply 75 287 520 by 12 103 014. This results in a very large number of possible pairings (9.11×10^{14}) forming the basis of the distribution of the difference between two sample means. It is the mean and the variance of this distribution that we are interested in.

Before going any further we need to introduce some notation. The notation given in Table 11.1 uses the subscripts 1 and 2 to indicate the population to which we are referring. As usual, we use Greek letters when referring to populations and Roman letters when referring to samples taken from the populations. The populations may be of different sizes, and so the samples may also be of different sizes.

Table 11.1 Notation used when dealing with two samples from two populations.

Population	Population parameters			Sample statistics		
	Size	Mean	Variance	Size	Mean	Variance
One	N_1	μ_1	σ_1^2	n_1	$\bar{x}_1$	s_1^2
Two	N_2	μ_2	σ_2^2	n_2	$\bar{x}_2$	s_2^2

The difference between the two population means is denoted by $\mu_1 - \mu_2$ and the difference between the two sample means by $\bar{x}_1 - \bar{x}_2$. The mean for the distribution of the difference between two sample means is denoted by $\mu_{\bar{x}_1 - \bar{x}_2}$ and the standard deviation by $\sigma_{\bar{x}_1 - \bar{x}_2}$. It may be shown that:

$$\mu_{\bar{x}_1 - \bar{x}_2} = \mu_1 - \mu_2$$

$$\sigma_{\bar{x}_1 - \bar{x}_2} = \sqrt{\frac{\sigma_1^2}{n_1} + \frac{\sigma_2^2}{n_2}}$$

At this stage we need to consider whether the samples are large ($n \geq 30$) or small ($n < 30$).

Differences between means of large samples

If both samples are large we do not need to assume that the distributions are normal and that the sample variances s_1^2 and s_2^2 will be good estimators of their respective population variances, and we can obtain a test statistic using the z-distribution from the formula

$$z = \frac{(\bar{x}_1 - \bar{x}_2) - (\mu_1 - \mu_2)}{\sqrt{\dfrac{s_1^2}{n_1} + \dfrac{s_2^2}{n_2}}}$$

The value obtained from this formula is then compared to a critical z-value read from the z-tables. If the obtained z-value is beyond the critical value then the null hypothesis is rejected. The null hypothesis usually states that there is no difference between the two sample means, and is written as

$$H_0 : \quad \mu_1 = \mu_2 \text{ or } H_0 : \quad \mu_1 - \mu_2 = 0$$

EXAMPLE 11.2

It has been claimed that, in the 20 – 24 age group, males have a higher mean systolic blood pressure than females. Independent random samples of males and females were selected and data pertaining to systolic blood pressure readings were obtained and are as follows:

Results	Males:	$n_1 = 31,$	$\bar{x}_1 = 125,$	$s_1^2 = 193.21$
	Females:	$n_2 = 41,$	$\bar{x}_2 = 117,$	$s_2^2 = 146.41$

Test the claim that males have a higher mean systolic blood pressure than females for this particular age group at the 5% level of significance.

Solution
We state our hypotheses as follows:
$$H_0 : \quad \mu_1 = \mu_2 \quad \text{vs} \quad H_1 : \quad \mu_1 > \mu_2$$

For $\alpha = 0.05$, we have a critical z-value of $+1.645$

From the above data summary we have $z = \dfrac{(125 - 117) - 0}{\sqrt{\dfrac{193.21}{31} + \dfrac{146.41}{41}}} = 2.555$

Since the obtained z-value (2.555) is beyond the critical value (1.645) we can reject the null hypothesis and conclude that males have a higher mean systolic blood pressure than females for this particular age group.

Small independent samples

When the sample size is small, $(n < 30)$ we make either of two possible assumptions concerning the population variances: we assume either that the variances are equal or that they are not equal. If it is reasonable to assume that the population variances are equal then we can estimate this common variance by calculating a *pooled estimate* using the sample variances as follows:

$$s_p^2 = \frac{(n_1 - 1)s_1^2 + (n_2 - 1)s_2^2}{n_1 + n_2 - 2}$$

The pooled estimate of the common variance s_p^2 is in fact a weighted average of the sample variances, with degrees of freedom being used as weightings. The test statistic we use is from the *t*-distribution because of the small sample sizes. The critical value is found from the *t*-tables using $n_1 + n_2 - 2$ degrees of freedom, and the *t*-value based upon the data is calculated using the following formula, where $s_p = \sqrt{s_p^2}$:

$$t = \frac{(\bar{x}_1 - \bar{x}_2) - (\mu_1 - \mu_2)}{s_p \sqrt{\dfrac{1}{n_1} + \dfrac{1}{n_2}}}$$

If the population variances cannot be assumed equal, we are limited to an approximate *t*-test because we can only approximate the degrees of freedom associated with $\sigma_{\bar{x}_1 - \bar{x}_2}$. This is best done using a computer package like Minitab.

Checking for equality of variances

To check that the population variances are equal, we divide the larger variance by the smaller variance and check to see how close the result is to the value one. This ratio of the variances is referred to as an *F-statistic* and is compared with a critical *F*-value obtained from the *F*-tables using $n_{lg} - 1$ degrees of freedom for the numerator and $n_{sm} - 1$ degrees of freedom for the denominator. (n_{lg} is the sample size associated with the sample having the larger variance, and n_{sm} is the sample size associated with the sample having the smaller variance.)

If the variances are approximately equal then the *F*-ratio will be close to one, so the larger the *F*-ratio the more likely that the variances are not the same. The hypotheses are written as

$$H_0: \quad \sigma_1^2 = \sigma_2^2 \quad \text{vs} \quad H_1: \quad \sigma_1^2 \neq \sigma_2^2$$

EXAMPLE 11.3

Experienced midwives have noticed that the more time a new born baby spends in the nursery the sooner the mother is likely to stop breastfeeding. This was investigated by taking a random sample of mothers who were still breastfeeding 6 weeks after the birth and noting the number of hours their babies had spent in the nursery. A similar sample was taken of mothers who were not breastfeeding 6 weeks after the birth of their babies. All mothers had normal deliveries and spent 5 days in hospital after giving birth. The number of hours spent by the babies in the nursery was as follows:

Breast-fed   52.8 57.6 52.8 60.0 55.2 40.8 62.4 43.2 50.4 52.8 57.6 45.6
Bottle-fed   67.2 74.4 72.0 79.2 69.6 74.4 64.8 69.6 76.8

Is there evidence here to suggest that babies still being breast-fed after 6 weeks spent less time in the nursery than babies currently being bottle-fed?

EXAMPLE **11.3** cont.

Breast-fed	Bottle-fed
$n_1 = 12$	$n_2 = 9$
$\bar{x}_1 = 52.6$	$\bar{x}_2 = 72.0$
$s_1 = 6.67$	$s_2 = 4.65$

Solution
1 State the hypotheses, choose a significance level and establish the critical value of the test statistic.

H_0: $\mu_1 = \mu_2$ (the average time spent in the nursery is the same for both goups of babies).
H_1: $\mu_1 < \mu_2$ (breast-fed babies spent less time in the nursery).

Use $\alpha = 0.05$ (Note one-tailed test).
Degrees of freedom = $n_1 + n_2 - 2 = 19$; so critical $t = -1.729$.

2. Check for equality of population variances.
H_0: $\sigma_1^2 = \sigma_2^2$ (variances are equal).
H_1: $\sigma_1^2 \neq \sigma_2^2$ (variances are not equal).

$$F = \frac{6.67^2}{4.65^2} = 2.06$$

For $\alpha = 0.05$, and df (11, 8) we find critical F between 3.28 and 3.35.

Since the calculated F-value is not beyond the critical F-value, we accept that the population variances are equal and use a pooled t-test.

3 Find the pooled estimate for the common variance.

$$s_p = \sqrt{\frac{(n_1-1)s_1^2 + (n_2-1)s_2^2}{n_1 + n_2 - 2}} = \sqrt{\frac{(11)44.49 + (8)21.62}{12 + 9 - 2}}$$

$$s_p = 5.904$$

4 Calculate the sample test statistic.

$$t = \frac{(\bar{x}_1 - \bar{x}_2) - (\mu_1 - \mu_2)}{s_p\sqrt{\frac{1}{n_1} + \frac{1}{n_2}}} = \frac{(52.6 - 72.0) - 0}{5.904\sqrt{\frac{1}{12} + \frac{1}{9}}} = -7.452$$

5 Finally draw a conclusion based upon the above observations.
Decision: Reject H_0 since the calculated t-value is beyond critical t.
Conclusion: Breast-fed babies spent significantly less time in the nursery than bottle-fed babies.

Using Minitab for independent samples

The Minitab printout below uses the data from Example 11.3. Note how the equality of the variances was tested, and how extra notes can be included in Minitab printouts by using either of the commands # or NOTE.

The obtained t-value of -7.45 can be compared with a critical t-value obtained from the t-tables, or the probability value $p = 0.00$ can be compared directly with the α-level. In this case we can reject H_0 because the p-value is less than the α-level. We conclude, as we did in Example 11.3, that the babies currently being breast-fed spent significantly less time in the hospital nursery than babies currently being bottle-fed. Note that Minitab prints out the pooled estimate of the standard deviation as well as a 95% confidence interval for the difference in the mean number of hours spent in the nursery for the two groups.

```
MTB > Desc C1 C2


             N      MEAN     MEDIAN     TRMEAN     STDEV     SEMEAN
breast      12      52.6       52.8       52.8      6.67       1.92
bottle       9      72.0       72.0       72.0      4.65       1.55


            MIN      MAX      Q1       Q3
breast     40.8     62.4     46.8     57.6
bottle     64.8     79.2     68.4     75.6

MTB > let K1=stdev(C1)**2/stdev(C2)**2
MTB > print k1
K1    2.05859
MTB > #This obtained F-statistic can be compared with a critical
MTB > #value by using the F-tables with 11 and 8 degrees of freedom.
MTB >
MTB > NOTE Alternatively, the probability of obtaining such an
        F-value
MTB > NOTE can be calculated by Minitab as follows:
MTB >
MTB > cdf k1;
SUBC> f 11 8.
  2.0586   0.8426
MTB > #The probability of an F-value beyond 2.0586 is 1 - 0.8426
MTB > #which is 0.1574. As this is greater than alpha = 0.05 we
MTB > #accept that the variances are the same.
MTB >
MTB > twos C1 C2;
SUBC> pooled;
SUBC> alt=-1.
TWOSAMPLE T FOR breast VS bottle
          N      MEAN     STDEV     SE MEAN
breast   12      52.6      6.67       1.9
bottle    9      72.0      4.65       1.5
95 PCT CI FOR MU breast - MU bottle: (-24.8, -14.0)
TTEST MU breast = MU bottle (VS LT): T= -7.45 P=0.0000 DF= 19
POOLED STDEV =     5.90
```

Figure 11.2 Minitab printout for data from Example 11.3.

Practical statistics for the health sciences

You can use both POOLED and ALTERNATIVE subcommands in either order. Simply end the first subcommand with a semicolon to indicate that another one is coming.

If there is evidence that the variances cannot be assumed to be equal, we simply omit the subcommand POOLED. In this case the resulting test is an approximate *t*-test. Figure 11.3 is a printout for the breast-fed/bottle-fed data assuming that variances are *not* equal. Compare this printout with Figure 11.2 (obtained using the subcommand POOLED) and note the slight differences that occur in the obtained *t*-value and the different values for the degrees of freedom and the confidence intervals. These values have been underlined for easier identification.

```
MTB > twos c1 c2

TWOSAMPLE T FOR breast VS bottle
             N      MEAN     STDEV     SE MEAN
breast      12      52.6     6.67        1.9
bottle       9      72.0     4.65        1.5
95 PCT CI FOR MU breast - MU bottle: (-24.6, -14.2)
TTEST MU breast = MU bottle (VS LT): T= -7.85 P=0.0000 DF= 18
```

Figure 11.3 Section of Minitab printout for data from Example 11.3, assuming that variances are not equal.

1   A physician employed by a large corporation believes that, due to an increase in sedentary life styles in the past decade, middle-aged men have become fatter. In 1980 the corporation measured the amount of body fat in their employees. For middle-aged men the scores were normally distributed with a mean of 18%. To test her hypothesis, the physician measured the fat percentage in a random sample of 12 middle-aged men employed by the corporation. The fat percentages found were as follows:

21, 16, 24, 28, 18, 20, 22, 22, 19, 25, 20, 27.

Can we conclude that middle-aged men employed by the corporation have become fatter? Use $\alpha = 0.05$ to test this theory.

2   You are interested in determining if an experimental birth-control pill has the side effect of changing blood pressure. You randomly sample 10 women from the city in which you live. You give five of them a placebo for a month and then measure their blood pressure. Then you switch them to the birth-control pill for a month and again measure their blood pressure. The other five women receive the same treatment except they are given the birth-control pill first for a month followed by the placebo for a month. The blood pressure readings are shown below. (To safeguard the women from unwanted pregnancy, another means of birth control which does not interact with the pill was used for the duration of the experiment.) Assume that the data are normal.

Subject	1	2	3	4	5	6	7	8	9	10
Pill	108	76	69	78	74	85	79	78	80	81
Placebo	102	68	66	71	76	80	82	79	78	85

(a) What is the alternative hypothesis? Assume a non-directional hypothesis is appropriate.
(b) What is the null hypothesis?
(c) What do you conclude? Use $\alpha = 0.01$.

3   A nurse was hired by a government environment agency to investigate the impact of a lead smelter on the level of lead in the blood of children living near the smelter. Ten children were chosen at random from those living near the smelter. A comparison group of seven children were randomly selected from those living in an area relatively free from possible lead pollution.

Blood samples were taken from the children and lead levels were determined. The following are the results (scores are in micrograms of lead per 100 mL of blood). Using $\alpha = 0.01$, what do you conclude?

Near   18, 16, 21, 14, 17, 19, 22, 24, 15
Not Near 9, 13, 8, 15, 17, 12, 11

4   A local business school claims that their graduates get higher-paying jobs than the national average. Last year's figures for salaries paid to all business school graduates on their first job showed a mean of $11.20 per hour. A random sample of 10 graduates from last year's class of the local business school showed the following hourly salaries for their first job:

$10.40, $11.30, $12.20, $11.80, $11.40, $10.70, $10.80, $11.60, $11.70, $11.90.

Evaluate the claim regarding the salaries of the local business school graduates using $\alpha = 0.05$.

5   As the principal of a private secondary school you are interested in finding out how the training in mathematics at your school compares with that of the public schools in your area. For the last 5 years the public schools have given graduating students a mathematics proficiency test. The distribution of scores has a mean of 78. You give all graduating students at your school the same mathematics proficiency test. The resulting distribution of 41 scores show a mean of 83 and a standard deviation of 12.2.

(a) What is the alternative hypothesis?
(b) What is the null hypothesis?
(c) Using $\alpha = 0.05$, what do you conclude?

6   The manager of the cosmetics section of a large department store wants to determine whether newspaper advertising really does increase sales. For her experiment she randomly selects 15 items currently in stock and proceeds to establish a baseline. The 15 items are priced at their usual competitive values, and the quantity of each item sold in a 1-week period is recorded. Then, without changing their price, she places a large advertisement in the newspaper for the 15 items. Again she records the quantity sold in a 1-week period. The results are shown below:

Item	1	2	3	4	5	6	7	8
Before	25	18	3	42	16	20	23	32
After	32	24	7	40	19	25	23	35

Item	9	10	11	12	13	14	15
Before	60	40	27	7	13	23	16
After	65	43	28	11	12	32	28

Using $\alpha = 0.05$, what do you conclude?

7 On the basis of her experience with clients, a clinical psychologist thinks that depression may interfere with sleep. She decides to test this idea. The sleep of nine depressed patients and eight normal controls is monitored for three successive nights. The average number of hours slept by each subject during the last two nights is shown below:

Hours of sleep
Depressed   9.2 7.5 3.9 7.1 6.1 6.6 7.4 7.4 5.9
Control   6.7 6.9 9.5 6.8 7.4 8.2 9.2 6.6

Is the clinician correct? Use $\alpha = 0.05$ in making your decision.

8 A random sample of $n_1 = 25$ taken from a normal population with standard deviation $\sigma_1 = 5.2$ has a mean $\bar{x}_1 = 81$. A second random sample of size $n_2 = 36$, taken from a different normal population with standard deviation $\sigma_2 = 3.4$, has a mean $\bar{x}_2 = 76$. Test the hypothesis $\mu_1 = \mu_2$ against the alternative $\mu_1 \neq \mu_2$. State a p-value in your conclusion.

9 To find out whether a new serum will arrest leukemia, nine mice which have reached an advanced stage of the disease are selected. Five mice receive the treatment and four do not. The survival times in months from the time the experiment commenced are as follows:

Treatment   2.1, 5.3, 1.4, 4.6, 0.9
No Treatment   1.9, 0.5, 2.8, 3.1

At the 0.05 level of significance, can the serum be said to be effective? Assume the two distributions to be normal, with equal variances.

10 The following data represent the times taken (in minutes) to perform two different operations.

Op.A 102, 86, 98, 109,   92
Op.B   81, 165, 97, 134, 92, 87, 114

Test the hypothesis that the average time taken for operation A is ten minutes less than that taken for operation B. Use a 1% level of significance and assume the distribution of times to be normal.

11 A test was conducted on a fleet of ambulances to determine whether the use of radial tyres instead of regular tyres improves fuel economy. Twelve ambulances were equipped with radial tyres and driven over a prescribed test course. Without changing drivers, the same vehicles were equipped with regular belted tyres and driven once again over the test course. Fuel consumption in kilometres/litre was recorded as follows:

Vehicle	Radial tyres	Belted tyres
1	8.4	8.2
2	9.4	9.8
3	13.2	12.4
4	14.0	13.8
5	13.4	13.6
6	9.0	8.8
7	10.4	11.4
8	12.0	11.6
9	14.8	13.8
10	9.8	9.4
11	12.2	12.0
12	10.4	9.8

At the 0.025 level of significance, can we conclude that ambulances equipped with radial tyres give better fuel economy than those equipped with belted tyres? Assume the populations to be normally distributed.

12 In both a professional nursing unit and a general ward, 14 patients suffering from diabetes were observed as part of a total nursing audit. The mean score for the professional unit was 156 with standard deviation 12.5, while the mean score for the general unit was 127 with standard deviation 14. Do these results suggest that there is a significant difference in the quality of the care experienced by these patients?

CHAPTER TWELVE

Distribution-free tests

LEARNING OBJECTIVES

After reading this chapter you should be able to:
- use an approximation to the sign test for paired or categorical data;
- apply the sign test by using binomial probability;
- use Minitab to evaluate a sign test;
- rank data from lowest to highest, including dealing with equal data values;
- calculate the critical statistic for the Wilcoxon signed-ranks test and use tables to check the critical values for the test;
- use and interpret the output of the Minitab command wtest;
- perform the appropriate calculation needed to calculate the test statistic for a Mann–Whitney test;
- use and interpret the output of the Minitab command mann; and
- know when it is appropriate to use a distribution-free test rather than a distribution-based test.

The Central Limit Theorem allows us to use the normal distribution to calculate the probability of obtaining a certain sample mean or more extreme values of the statistic if the sample size is large (>30) or if the population from which the sample is taken can be assumed to be normal. Unfortunately our data do not always meet these criteria. Not only may we have small samples taken from skewed populations, but the data may well be nominal or ordinal. In the latter case it is not appropriate to calculate means, standard deviations and so on. This implies that the techniques used in the previous chapters are not applicable and that other procedures must be developed in order to make estimations and test hypotheses for variables of this nature. These alternative procedures are known collectively as *distribution-free tests* or *non-parametric tests*.

Distribution-free tests are so named because they do not depend upon assumptions involving the shape of the population distribution. They may be used for either nominal or ranked data. They may also be used in place of the usual parametric tests when such tests require extensive calculation of means and variances. Distribution-free tests are not as powerful as their counterparts that make use of the Central Limit Theorem, but they are often very quick and easy to carry out, particularly when you are initially exploring the data.

12.1   The sign test

The simplest of all distribution-free tests is the *sign test*, which considers only the number of *positive* or *negative* signs. It is suitable for single-sample experiments, or two-sample experiments where there is a basis for pairing the results for each group and calculating difference scores, as in a repeated measures design. The sign test can be used in any situation where the null hypothesis specifies that either one of two possibilities is equally likely. It is to these possibilities that we allocate plus or minus signs. For example, we can test if the median is equal to some value k. *Positive* signs are assigned to data values greater than k and *negative* signs to those values less than k. Values equal to k are not included in the calculation. According to the null hypothesis, if the median is in fact equal to k we would expect the same number of data values above the median as below. Therefore the sign test is based upon a binomial probability distribution with $p = 0.5$. Example 12.1 illustrates a test of the median being equal to some claimed value k; the important point to note is the exclusion of data values that equal k.

EXAMPLE 12.1

It is often claimed that the sale of houses is a good indicator of movement in the economy. Last month the median price of houses sold in country areas was $85 000. A survey was taken of houses sold during this last week and the following information was collected:

Sale Prices	$ 67 500	$79 950	$95 700	$ 85 000	$90 000	$89 950	$125 750
	$145 000	$87 500	$92 000	$156 000	$82 500	$88 750	$ 97 500

Is there evidence to suggest that the median sale price has shifted significantly from that obtained last month? Test at the 5% level of significance.

Practical statistics for the health sciences

Solution

In this case we have one example where the sale price was equal to last month's median price of $85 000. This value cannot be given a plus or a minus sign, so it is excluded from the data. We now have a reduced sample size of 13 sale prices, three of which are below the median value of $85 000. The following summary applies:

$n = 13$, 10 positives, 3 negatives, $\alpha = 0.05$

H_0 : Median house price has not changed from last month.

H_1 : Median house price has increased significantly.

The test statistic is $\Pr(x \geq 10)$, and from the binomial tables ($n = 13$, $p = 0.5$) we have $\Pr(x \geq 10) = 0.0037$

Conclusion

As the probability (0.0037) is less than the chosen α-level we can reject H_0 and conclude that the recent median sale price for houses in the area has increased compared to the previous month.

Note that the above example was a one-tailed test. If a two-tailed test was required then the p-value obtained above would have been doubled. The same result would also have been obtained had we calculated the probability $\Pr(x \leq 3)$. Therefore it makes no difference whether you deal with the positives or the negatives, because the binomial distribution with $p = 0.5$ is symmetrical. The following steps provide a basic outline of a sign test:

1 Designate each sample value as either a *plus* (+) or *minus* (−)

2 Count the number of plus signs.

3 Use the binomial distribution to calculate $\Pr(X \geq x \text{ plus signs})$ from the binomial tables where n = sample size, $p = 0.5$, x = no. of + values or − values.

4 If the resulting probability is less than the chosen α-level, reject H_0.

The sign test for matched pairs

When dealing with paired data that is not normal, the sign test is often a quick and easy test to use. The numbers themselves are ignored, and consideration is only given as to whether the *differences* between the pairs of data values are positive or negative. Each difference score is designated as a plus or a minus, and we proceed to use the binomial distribution to calculate the probability of obtaining the number of plus signs achieved.

EXAMPLE 12.2

The safety officer at a particular hospital was concerned at the number of staff injuries in the main work areas of the hospital. A safety awareness program was undertaken by all staff. To ascertain the effectiveness of the program the number of injuries to nursing staff in nine different work areas in the hospital was noted for the three months preceding the safety awareness program and for the three months immediately following the program. Based upon the data

EXAMPLE   12.2   cont.

below, what can the safety officer conclude?

Total injuries per three months in nine work areas
Before	22	11	13	5	7	10	9	8	8
After	17	9	14	4	2	8	11	6	7

Solution

H_0:   The safety program has had no effect. ie $\eta_B = \eta_A$
H_1:   The safety program has been effective. ie $\eta_B > \eta_A$

From the data above we see that seven of the nine work areas recorded a decrease in the number of injuries *after* the safety program. The test statistic is therefore

$\Pr(x \geq 7) = 0.0899$

As this value is greater than $\alpha = 0.05$, we fail to reject H_0 and conclude that the safety program has not had a significant effect.

The conclusion reached in the example above may appear somewhat surprising given that reductions were recorded in seven of the nine work areas, and in some cases the reductions seemed to be considerable. The sign test, however, does not take into consideration the *magnitude* of any reduction, only whether or not a reduction occurred. It only considers whether sample values lie above or below the median and ignores how far these values are from the median. In this sense it is not as powerful as the paired t-test which uses more information from the difference scores. But it is a quick and easy test that has the advantage of being applicable to dichotomous data that cannot be recorded on a numerical scale but can be represented by positive and negative responses. We need make no assumptions about the underlying population, and no complicated calculations are necessary.

The sign test for categorical data

The sign test can also be used when measurements are not numerical and there are two categories. In this case we are primarily interested in whether or not our sample indicates a preference for one category or the other. If we assume that there is no preference, we would expect a similar number of values in each category. This situation can also be modelled by the binomial distribution with n = sample size and $p = 0.5$.

EXAMPLE   12.3

A class of 20 students was asked to indicate their preferences for either one of two similarly priced holiday packages. The results were as follows:

Europe	West Coast USA
4	16

Is there evidence to suggest that there is a preference for one holiday destination over the other?

EXAMPLE   12.3   cont.

Solution
We state the hypotheses as

H_0 :   There is no significant difference in the preferences.
H_1 :   Significantly more students prefer West Coast USA.

We choose an α-level of 0.05. The probability of getting the above result (or one just as extreme) is equivalent to finding $\Pr(x \geq 16)$, where x represents the number of students who prefer the West Coast USA holiday.

From the binomial tables with $n = 20$ and $p = 0.5$ we find that $\Pr(x \geq 16) = 0.006$. This value is the test statistic and is compared with the chosen α-level.

Conclusion
We reject H_0 because the obtained probability (0.006) is less than the chosen α-level (0.05). We conclude that there is a significant difference in preference between the two holiday packages.

An approximation to the sign test

If the null hypothesis is true we would expect half of the observed signs to be positive and half to be negative. That is, the expected number of + signs would be $0.5n$. For the *discrepancy* between the 'observed' number of + signs and the 'expected' number ($0.5n$), the following approximations are a reasonable guide:

- a discrepancy $\sqrt{n}$ is significant at the 5% level,
- a discrepancy $1.3\sqrt{n}$ is significant at the 1% level,
- a discrepancy $1.67\sqrt{n}$ is significant at 0.1% level.

Using Minitab to perform a sign test

Minitab can be used to perform a sign test as long as the data can be put into one or two columns. Figure 12.1 shows the Minitab analyses for both the single-sample and the paired-samples tests considered in Examples 12.1 and 12.2. For the first case notice that the value for the median claimed by the null hypothesis ($\eta = 85000$) appears in the main command line. In the second case, notice that for the paired data the difference scores in column 4 were obtained in such a way that, if the After scores were less than the Before scores, these decreases appear as negative values in column 4. This was achieved by subtracting the column 2 values from the column 3 values.

```
CASE 1:
MTB > set c1
DATA> 67500 79950 95700 85000 90000 89950 125750 145000 87500 92000
DATA> 156000 82500 88750 97500
DATA> end
MTB > stest 85000 c1;
SUBC> alt -1 .

SIGN TEST OF MEDIAN = 85000 VERSUS G.T. 85000

          N    BELOW   EQUAL    ABOVE    P-VALUE   MEDIAN
C1       14        3       1       10     0.0037   -5.000
```

```
CASE 2:
MTB > set C2
MTB > 22 11 13 5 7 10 9 8 8
DATA > set c3
DATA > 17 9 14 4 2 8 11 6 7
DATA > end
MTB > name c2 'before' c3 'after'
MTB > let c4=c3-c2
MTB > print c4
C4
 -5  -2  +1  -1  -5  -2  2  -2  -1
MTB > stest c4;
SUBC> alte = -1.

SIGN TEST OF MEDIAN = 0.00000 VERSUS L.T. 0.00000

        N    BELOW   EQUAL   ABOVE   P-VALUE   MEDIAN
C4      9      7       0       2      0.0898   -2.000
MTB > cdf;
SUBC> binomial 9 0.5.

 BINOMIAL WITH N =  9 P = 0.500000
   K P( X LESS OR = K)
   0      0.0020
   1      0.0195
   2      0.0898
   3      0.2539
   4      0.5000
   5      0.7461
   6      0.9102
   7      0.9805
   8      0.9980
   9      1.0000
```

Figure 12.1 Minitab printout for single-sample and paired-samples tests in Examples 12.1 and 12.2.

Note that the obtained probability value of 0.0898 in the second case can also be found using the cumulative binomial probabilities obtained from Minitab using the CDF command. This table gives the probabilities for $x \leq k$, hence

$$Pr(7 \text{ or more decreases}) = Pr(2 \text{ or less increases})$$

It is the latter probability that we look up in the table. This is the probability that has been underlined in the printout in Figure 12.1.

12.2   The Wilcoxon signed-ranks test

The Wilcoxon signed-ranks test (or Wilcoxon T-test) can be used to analyse the results of experiments where we can *rank* the difference scores obtained from the raw data. Difference scores can be found either by subtracting paired data values from each other or by calculating the differences between a set of obtained values and a claimed value for a median. It is a more powerful test than the sign test

Practical statistics for the health sciences

because it considers the *magnitudes* of these differences between paired values or deviations from a claimed median.

The null hypothesis usually claims that the median of the difference scores is zero (ie the variable of interest has had no effect) or that the median is equal to some value k. The alternative hypothesis claims that there has been some effect. In this test the absolute values of the difference scores (or deviations from some hypothesised median) are ranked from smallest to largest. The smallest difference gets a rank of 1, the next smallest a rank of 2, and so on. If two or more difference scores have the same absolute values, each is assigned the average of the ranks they would have otherwise occupied. Zero difference scores are ignored. The following steps outline the procedure for the Wilcoxon signed-ranks test:

1 Calculate differences (ignoring zero differences).

2 Rank the differences, from the smallest (rank = 1) to the largest, ignoring the signs.

3 Sum the negative ranks ($\Sigma R-$) and the positive ranks ($\Sigma R+$).

4 The test statistic T is the lesser of the two values $\Sigma R-$ and $\Sigma R+$, and is compared to a critical value obtained from the appropriate set of tables.

If the null hypothesis is true we would expect the same spread of scores above and below the median, and the sum of the positive ranks would be equal (or very nearly so) to the sum of the negative ranks. The larger the difference between $\Sigma R-$ and $\Sigma R+$ the more likely it will be that H_0 is false.

EXAMPLE **12.4**

Many enthusiastic supporters of orientation activities would cite 'more positive attitude towards studies' as one of the benefits for participating students. A group of students was surveyed prior to a 5-day orientation program. They were given a questionnaire which measured attitude towards tertiary study using a 50-point scale. The higher the points, the more favourable the attitude towards tertiary study. A similar questionnaire was given to the students after the orientation program. Ten students were selected at random, and their scores before and after the program were recorded.

Attitude score

Before	40	33	36	34	40	31	30	36	24	20
After	44	40	49	36	39	40	27	42	35	28

Is there evidence to suggest that the orientation program had a positive effect on attitude towards tertiary study for this sample of students? Test at the 5% level.

Solution

H_0: The orientation program had no effect on student attitudes.

H_1: The program had a positive effect on student attitudes.

Construct a table of difference scores:

Before	40	33	36	34	40	31	30	36	24	20
After	44	40	49	36	39	40	27	42	35	28
Differences	4	7	13	2	−1	9	−3	6	11	8
Ranked Differences	4	6	10	2	1	8	3	5	9	7
Signed Ranks	4	6	10	2	−1	8	−3	5	9	7

EXAMPLE **12.4**   **cont.**

From this table we obtain $\Sigma R- = 4$ and $\Sigma R+ = 51$. Our test statistic is therefore $T = 4$.

From the tables for Wilcoxon's T we find the critical value of T to be 11. We can therefore reject H_0 at the 5% level and conclude that the orientation program had a positive effect on the attitudes of students towards their tertiary studies.

Using Minitab to perform a Wilcoxon signed-ranks test

If the data above are entered into columns 1 and 2 and the difference scores put into column 3, the appropriate command for the Wilcoxon signed-ranks test is WTEST c3. The p-value of 0.010 is less than $\alpha = 0.05$ so H_0 is rejected, as it was in the manual analysis above. An approximate 95% confidence interval (94.7%) for the median was obtained using the command WINT. Again, by testing that the median equals zero we are in fact testing that half the ranks will be negative and half will be positive, thus resulting in the median rank being equal to zero. Notice also in the printout in Figure 12.2 that Minitab uses the larger of the two values $\Sigma R-$ and $\Sigma R+$ and calculates the probability of obtaining a result as extreme as, or more extreme than, that obtained from the data. With Minitab the obtained p-value is compared to the chosen α-level.

```
MTB > let c3=c2-c1
MTB > name c3 'Diffnce'
MTB > print c3

Diffnce
   4    7   13    2   -1    9   -3    6   11    8

MTB > wtest c3;
SUBC> alt=+1.

TEST OF MEDIAN = 0.000000 VERSUS MEDIAN G.T.  0.000000

                    N FOR      WILCOXON                 ESTIMATED
              N     TEST       STATISTIC    P-VALUE      MEDIAN
Diffnce      10      10          51.0        0.010       6.000
MTB > wint c3

              ESTIMATED    ACHIEVED
              N     MEDIAN   CONFIDENCE   CONFIDENCE INTERVAL
Diffnce      10      6.00      94.7        (  2.00,   9.50)
```

Figure 12.2 Minitab printout for a Wilcoxon signed-ranks test on the data from Example 12.4.

The data on hospital staff injuries used in Example 12.2 is analysed in Example 12.5 using the Wilcoxon signed-ranks test.

EXAMPLE 12.5

Recall that the number of accidents before and after the safety awareness program were put into columns 1 and 2, with the difference scores in column 3 (C2 – C1).

We test to see if Before is better than After.

H_0 : The program had no effect (ie $\eta_{Diff} = 0$).

H_1 : The program was effective (ie $\eta_{Diff} < 0$).

```
MTB > wtest c3;
SUBC> alt=-1.

TEST OF MEDIAN = 0.000000 VERSUS MEDIAN L.T.  0.000000

                        N FOR    WILCOXON                ESTIMATED
               N        TEST     STATISTIC   P-VALUE      MEDIAN
Difference     9         9          7.5       0.043        -1.5
```

We see from the printout that the obtained p-value is 0.043. As this is less than $\alpha = 0.05$ we can reject H_0 and conclude that there is sufficient evidence to suggest that the safety awareness program has been effective in reducing the number of accidents. Note that the sign test was not able to reject H_0 in this instance, because it gave a p-value of 0.0898. The smaller p-value obtained by the Wilcoxon test allows us to reject the null hypothesis. We now proceed to find a suitable confidence interval based on our sample data.

```
MTB > wint c4
                 ESTIMATED     ACHIEVED
            N      MEDIAN     CONFIDENCE    CONFIDENCE INTERVAL
Total       9      -1.50        95.6          ( -3.5,  0.00 )
```

The Wilcoxon confidence interval is not an exact 95% confidence interval. The case above is interesting because the interval actually has the value 0.00 as one of its boundaries. This is not all that surprising given the closeness of the p-value (0.043) to the α-level of 5%.

12.3   The Mann–Whitney test

An appropriate test to use when comparing the means or medians of two independent samples from non-normal distributions is the Mann–Whitney test. This test is also sometimes referred to as the Wilcoxon ranked-sum test, not to be confused with the Wilcoxon signed-ranks test described in the previous section.

The Mann–Whitney test measures the degree of separation between two samples by considering the *ranks* of each of the observations considered as a *combined group*. For two samples of size n_1 and n_2, we assign ranks so that the smallest value of the *combined data set* receives a ranking of 1, the next smallest a ranking of 2, and so on up to the largest value. If two or more of the data values are tied, each is assigned the *average* of the ranks they would have received had there been no ties. This is the same procedure as that followed in the Wilcoxon signed-ranks test. The test statistic is defined as

W = sum of the ranks of the *first* (ie smaller) sample.

This value is then compared to a critical value obtained from the appropriate tables.

The null hypothesis assumes that the two populations from which the samples were drawn have the same distribution. The alternative hypothesis assumes that one population has a different mean or median than the other. If the two samples come from populations with the same distributions, or from the same population, the total of the ranks of the two samples should be roughly the same, depending on the relative sample sizes. The two totals will be quite different if the samples have come from populations with different means or medians. A very high or very low value of W indicates that the samples come from populations with different locations.

An illustration of the concept involved here can be seen in the representation of the two samples by x's and o's plotted on a number line.

```
              x   x   x   x   x   x   o   x   x  ox  o   o  oo  o   o   o   o  oo
Case 1    |___|___|___|___|___|___|___|___|___|___|___|___|___|___|___|___|___|___|___|___|
```

The two samples are clearly different and it is unlikely that they could be drawn from the same population. The x's would receive lower rankings than the o's.

```
              x   o   x  ox  x   o   o   x   o   x   o   x  oo  xx  o   x   o  xo
Case 2    |___|___|___|___|___|___|___|___|___|___|___|___|___|___|___|___|___|___|___|___|
```

Each sample in this second case occupies a similar range on the number line. The sample values (the x's and o's) are well mixed, and most likely could have been drawn from populations having the same distribution.

In Case 1 the null hypothesis would probably be rejected because the sum of the rankings for the sample of x's would be considerably lower than that for the o's. In Case 2 H_0 would not be rejected because the sum of the rankings for each sample would be nearly the same.

EXAMPLE 12.6

The managers at a particular hospital were concerned about apparent differences in the efficiency of nursing staff in the children's ward of the hospital. In particular they were interested in the differences between staff rostered in the mornings and those in the afternoons. Independent random samples of eight morning staff and seven afternoon staff were chosen, and the time taken to complete a specified task was noted for each. Is there evidence to suggest that there is a difference between the two groups of staff?

Morning Shift   6, 5, 5, 4, 0, 2, 1, 1
Afternoon Shift   8, 3, 7, 14, 9, 12, 16

We have two independent samples of sizes $n_1 = 8$ and $n_2 = 7$, and we cannot assume that the data is normally distributed; in this case it appears to be positively skewed, so a Mann–Whitney test is appropriate.

Solution

H_0: There is no difference between the shifts; $\eta_1 = \eta_2$

H_1: There is a difference between the two shifts; $\eta_1 \neq \eta_2$

EXAMPLE 12.6   cont.

First the scores are combined and ranked accordingly:

	Morning Shift								Afternoon Shift					
	6	5	5	4	0	2	1	1	8	3	7	14	9	12	16
Ranks	9	$7\frac{1}{2}$	$7\frac{1}{2}$	6	1	4	$2\frac{1}{2}$	$2\frac{1}{2}$	11	5	10	14	12	13	15
Sum Ranks				40								80			

The test statistic $W = 80$ is the sum of the ranks for the afternoon shift (the smaller sample). From the tables, samples of sizes 7 and 8 give the upper critical value $W_t = 73$.

Conclusion

$W = 80$ is beyond $W_t = 71$ so we can reject H_0 in favour of H_1.

There was a significant difference in the time taken to complete the specified task. It seems that staff on the morning shift took less time to complete the specified task than staff from the afternoon shift.

Note that in Example 12.6 we used the upper critical value from the Mann–Whitney tables. This was because the sum of the ranks from the smaller sample was in fact greater than the sum of the ranks from the larger sample. The following outline summarises the steps required for the Mann–Whitney test.

1 State your null hypothesis: H_0:   median of group 1 = median of group 2.

2 Decide on an appropriate alternative hypothesis, ie

H_1:   median of group 1 ≠ median of group 2
or
median of group 1 > median of group 2
or
median of group 1 < median of group 2

3 Choose an appropriate α-level.

4 Look up the critical value(s) from the tables using the sample sizes given.

5 Assign ranks to the data in increasing order. For tied scores, average the ranks.

6 Calculate the sum of the ranks associated with the smaller sample.

7 Compare with the critical values, and accept H_0 if the test statistic is *within* the tabulated values.

8 State a conclusion in words.

Using Minitab to perform a Mann–Whitney test

The Minitab printout below shows the output generated by the command MANN for the data in Example 12.6. The morning shift data was stored in column 1 and the afternoon shift data in column 2. The printout for the Mann–Whitney test is a little different from previous Minitab hypothesis test printouts, and there are several points worthy of note.

(a) The test statistic is given as $W = 40$. This value is in fact the sum of the ranks associated with the morning shift data, because it was mentioned first in the command.

(b) The median for the first column mentioned is referred to as ETA1, and for the second column, ETA2.

(c) The value (at the end) at which the test is said to be significant is the p-value. This is usually easier to use as the basis for testing H_0.

(d) In order to accept H_0, the confidence interval for the difference between the medians should contain 0, because if the two groups were similar the difference between their respective medians would be close to zero.

(e) If a one-tail test is required, the direction of the test is indicated using ALT=±1 on the main command line rather than as a subcommand. For example, the command MANN ALT=1 c2 c1 would perform a one-tail test to test if the median from the data in column 2 is *greater than* that from column 1. In that case the median time taken by the afternoon shift would be greater than that of the morning shift.

```
MTB > mann c1 c2

Mann-Whitney Confidence Interval and Test

am     N = 8    Median =    3.000
pm     N = 7    Median =    9.000
Point estimate for ETA1-ETA2 is   -7.000
95.7 pct c.i. for ETA1-ETA2 is (-11.001, -1.997)
W = 40.0
Test of ETA1 = ETA2 vs. ETA1 n.e. ETA2 is significant at 0.0065
The test is significant at 0.0064 (adjusted for ties)

MTB > mann alt=1 c2 c1

Mann-Whitney Confidence Interval and Test

pm     N = 7    Median =    9.000
am     N = 8    Median =    3.000
Point estimate for ETA1-ETA2 is    7.000
95.7 pct c.i. for ETA1-ETA2 is (1.997,11.001)
W = 80.0
Test of ETA1 = ETA2 vs. ETA1 g.t. ETA2 is significant at 0.0033
The test is significant at 0.0032 (adjusted for ties)
```

Figure 12.3 Minitab printout for Mann–Whitney test on the data from Example 12.6.

Notice from the printout how the test statistic W changes according to which column is mentioned first, and that the p-value has been halved for the one-tail test.

Practical statistics for the health sciences

12.4 Distribution-free versus distribution-based procedures

Since distribution-based procedures generally use more of the information available in a sample, it is not surprising that, correctly applied, they are usually more efficient than comparable distribution-free procedures. That is, either greater precision is achieved for a given sample size or, equivalently, a smaller sample is required for some specified precision.

When sampling from paired normal populations, the sign test is about half as efficient as the t-test for paired differences. The Mann–Whitney test is only marginally less efficient (92–95%) than the t-test for independent samples.

On the other hand, however, distribution-free procedures are often very easy to work with. Their respective test statistics are simple to compute and do not depend on a knowledge of an underlying distribution for their validity. In a distribution-based procedure, departures from the assumed population model may well render any conclusions suspect.

1   An international breakfast food company is considering an expense-free holiday for its senior executives. In order to determine preference for a week in Fiji or a week in Bali a random sample of 18 executives was asked their preference. Four chose Bali and 14 chose Fiji. Is this difference statistically significant?

2   A real estate agent suggests that the median selling price for houses in the local area is $85 000. A sample of 18 houses taken from a Saturday newspaper shows the following house prices:

$122 500	$115 000	$ 68 000	$35 000
$ 98 000	$ 89 950	$138 500	$69 950
$ 72 500	$ 82 000	$ 98 500	$58 000
$125 500	$129 950	$ 75 000	$68 000
$127 000	$123 500		

Use a sign test and $\alpha = 0.05$ to test the agent's claim.

3   Anxiety about statistics is perceived to be a common problem facing nursing students commencing studies in this area. To test the effectiveness of an anxiety-reduction workshop, seven students were given a test to measure their anxiety level. After completing the workshop, a follow-up test was administered. The pre-workshop and post-workshop test results are given below:

Pre-workshop   32 39 43 21 29 35 34
Post-workshop   30 31 44 21 26 36 28

Assuming that the scores have a symmetric distribution, test the hypothesis that the workshop reduced anxiety levels. (The lower the score, the lower the anxiety level.)

4   In the past, the number of defective syringes per lot of 1000 has had a median of 8. To test whether this is still the case, the number of defective syringes per lot of 1000 is monitored over a certain period. The number of defectives in the lots are:

3, 11, 6, 22, 9, 12, 11, 12, 7, 12, 8, 14, 10, 7, 6, 8, 16, 10, 13

Nursing staff believe the number of defectives has increased. Use a Wilcoxon signed-rank test to test this conjecture at the 0.05 level of significance.

5   An employee for a food processing plant notices a marked reduction in deterioration in unrefrigerated food which has been exposed to gamma radiation. She matches 10 food samples (labelled A to J) by type, quantity, degree of freshness and source, and exposes one of each pair, randomly selected, to the radiation. She then determines the deterioration rate of the foods over a period of 1 week during which all foods are stored as they normally would be. The deterioration rate is defined by an analysis of various factors, including retention of nutritive value, moisture, appealing appearance, and so forth. The results are shown here (unit = hundredths per week).

Pair	A	B	C	D	E	F	G	H	I	J
Not exposed	32	18	28	34	22	17	41	23	30	20
Exposed	19	21	21	17	24	12	24	28	18	10

Use the sign test and an $\alpha = 0.05$ level of significance to determine whether the radiation has in fact reduced the deterioration rate.

6   A psychologist gives a test to four male nurses and five female nurses to see if there is any significant difference (at $\alpha = 0.05$) in their test scores. The male nurses obtain scores of 23, 18, 22 and 21, and the female nurses obtain scores of 23, 28, 25, 24 and 26. Using a non-parametric technique, what conclusions might you draw from the study?

7   Two groups of nurses were given a questionnaire to ascertain their degree of job satisfaction. The scale ranged from 0 to 100. The groups were divided into those who had under 5 years of work experience and those who had 5 or more years of work experience. The data were as shown:

<5 Years 78, 98, 83, 86, 75, 77, 72, 68, 56, 93, 97
≥5 Years 94, 79, 82, 85, 73, 66, 64, 59, 2, 58, 63

At $\alpha = 0.10$, and assuming that the degree of job satisfaction has a symmetrical distribution, can you conclude that there is no difference in the job satisfaction of each group?

8   To test the effect of a health promotion film, students were randomly assigned to one of two

groups. Group 1 answered a questionnaire, while group 2 viewed the film and then answered the questionnaire. Higher scores indicated more positive attitudes towards healthier living.

Group 1 17, 31, 14, 12, 29, 7, 19, 28, 3
Group 2 10, 29, 37, 41, 16, 45, 34, 57

Do these results suggest that the film has had a significant positive effect?

9 The following data represent the time (in minutes) that a patient had to wait on 12 visits to a doctor's office before being seen by the doctor.

17, 15, 20, 20, 32, 28, 25, 35, 24, 12, 26, 25

Use both the sign test and the Wilcoxon signed-ranks test at the 5% level of significance to test the doctor's claim that the median waiting time for her patients is no more than 20 minutes. How do you explain the result?

10 It is claimed that a new diet will reduce a person's weight by 4.5 kg on average in a 3-week period. The weights of 10 people who followed the diet were recorded at the beginning and at the end of the diet program. The following results were obtained:

Subject	Weight before	Weight after
1	58.5	60.0
2	60.3	54.9
3	61.7	58.1
4	69.0	62.1
5	64.0	58.5
6	62.6	59.9
7	56.7	54.4
8	63.6	60.2
9	68.2	62.3
10	59.4	58.7

Test the hypothesis that the diet reduces the median weight by 4.5 kg against the alternative

hypothesis that the median difference in weight is less than 4.5 kg. Use a 5% level of significance.

11 The following figures represent the number of hours that two different types of calculators operate before a new battery is required.

Calculator A   5.5, 5.6, 6.3, 4.6, 5.3, 5.0, 6.2, 5.8, 5.1
Calculator B   3.8, 4.8, 4.3, 4.2, 4.0, 4.9, 4.5, 5.2, 4.5

Use a suitable test with $\alpha = 0.01$ to determine if calculator A operates longer than calculator B.

12 The number of prescriptions filled by two pharmacies over a 10-day period were as follows:

Pharmacy A   19, 21, 15, 17, 24, 12, 19, 14, 20, 18
Pharmacy B   17, 15, 12, 12, 16, 15, 11, 13, 14, 21

Use a suitable test to determine whether the two pharmacies, on average, fill the same number of prescriptions against the alternative that pharmacy A fills more prescriptions than pharmacy B.

13 The quality of record-keeping in a general ward and a professional nursing unit was assessed with the following results:

General unit   16, 18, 15, 19, 14, 17
Professional unit   19, 18, 18, 16, 19, 17, 20

Does the data indicate that there is a significant difference between the two groups of nurses? Test at the 5% level of significance.

14 The extent to which nursing staff taught the necessary procedures for their patients' independence in a general ward and a professional nursing unit was assessed with the following results:

General unit   21, 24, 30, 26, 26, 34, 15
Professional unit   30, 33, 29, 31, 28

Does this indicate that nurses from the professional unit are doing a more effective job? Test at the 5% level of significance.

13.1 Chi-square goodness of fit test

A method of testing whether frequencies we observe match with frequencies we expect, based on past experience or a theoretical model.

13.2 Chi-square test of independence (two variables)

A test that uses contingency tables for two variables; and a procedure for testing whether the two variables are independent.

CHAPTER THIRTEEN

Chi-square procedures

After reading this chapter you should be able to:
- write suitable hypotheses for a goodness of fit test;
- calculate expected frequencies based on theoretical models;
- correctly determine the degrees of freedom for each situation;
- evaluate the chi-square statistic for a set of expected and observed frequencies;
- write suitable hypotheses to test the independence of two variables;
- calculate expected frequencies based on the assumption that the null hypothesis (that the two variables are independent) is true; and
- correctly use and interpret the output of the Minitab command CHISQUARE.

A survey of Australian people in 1990 found that more than half (52.8%) did not have any private health insurance cover. The survey, of 8500 people, also showed a considerably higher proportion of single contributors (ie contributors with no dependent children) who did not have private health cover. These results are displayed below as pie graphs. The four categories were (a) no private cover, (b) hospital cover only, (c) ancillary cover only, and (d) both hospital and ancillary cover.

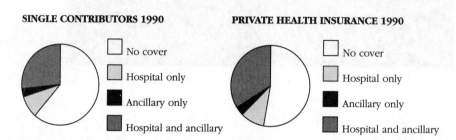

SINGLE CONTRIBUTORS 1990   PRIVATE HEALTH INSURANCE 1990

- No cover
- Hospital only
- Ancillary only
- Hospital and ancillary

Figure 13.1 Health insurance cover for (a) single contributors and (b) all contributors.

If we compare the pie graphs we can see that there is a difference between the single contributors and the population at large. However, can we say that there is a significant difference? Would another sample provide results that show less difference? This section deals with a method of determining whether or not there is a significant difference between the frequencies we might expect and the frequencies we actually observe. The statistical test that does this is called a *chi-square test*, and the test statistic is calculated using the following formula

$$\chi^2 = \sum \frac{(O-E)^2}{E}$$

where O is the observed frequency and E is the expected frequency. The value of this test statistic is compared to a critical value obtained from the tables of the chi-square distribution using the relevant degrees of freedom.

A chi-square test can be used to test whether or not a particular data set is similar to what was expected, or if two variables are dependent or independent. Instead of comparing actual scores as we do with z-tests and t-tests, we compare how often particular scores or categories occur. Since we are primarily concerned with only how many times each data item occurs, the data itself need not be of numeric scaling but may be nominal or categorical, as in the health insurance example. Observed frequencies are compared to the frequencies that would be expected if the null hypothesis were true. The calculated chi-square statistic represents a measure of difference between the observed and expected values.

13.1   Chi-square goodness of fit test

Chi-square *goodness of fit* tests are used to compare the composition of a sample with that of a theoretical distribution. It is in this sense that the test is often referred to as a goodness of fit test because we are evaluating how well the observed frequencies fit the expected frequencies, according to a stated null hypothesis. The null hypothesis for a chi-square goodness of fit test usually takes the form:

H_0: There is no significant difference between the pattern of data observed and that expected.

The alternative hypothesis states that there *is* a difference.

The chi-square goodness of fit hypothesis states that there *is* a significant difference.

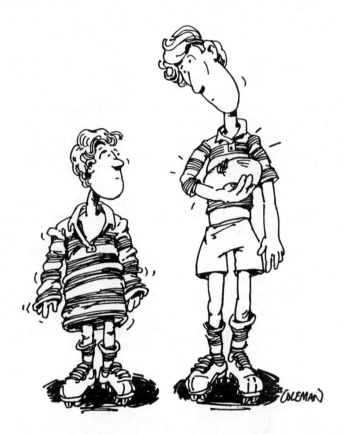

EXAMPLE 13.1

Suppose you are interested in determining whether there is a difference among student nurses in their preference for work experience in particular hospital wards. A random sample of 200 student nurses is selected and asked to indicate in which of the four wards listed they would prefer to work. The results are as follows:

Children's	Midwifery	Emergency	General
45	40	65	50

Solution

H_0: There is an equal preference for each of the areas.
H_1: There is not an equal preference for each of the areas.

EXAMPLE 13.1 cont.

As there are four categories there are three degrees of freedom associated with this test, so using an α-level of 5% implies that the critical value for the test statistic is $\chi^2 = 7.815$.

According to the null hypothesis we would expect equal numbers of student nurses to prefer working in each of the areas mentioned. Therefore the expected frequencies for each of the four areas is 50 ($\frac{1}{4}$ of the 200 sampled per category).

The calculated value for the test statistic is given by:

$$\chi^2 = \sum \frac{(O-E)^2}{E} = \frac{(45-50)^2}{50} + \frac{(40-50)^2}{50} + \frac{(65-50)^2}{50} + \frac{(50-50)^2}{50}$$

$$= \frac{25}{50} + \frac{100}{50} + \frac{225}{50} + \frac{0}{50} = 0.50 + 2.00 + 4.50 + 0 = 7.00$$

As the obtained value for the test statistic ($\chi^2 = 7.00$) is not beyond the critical value (7.815), we fail to reject H_0. There is not enough evidence to conclude that student nurses have a particular preference for working in any one of the wards mentioned. It would seem that they have an equal preference for each of the four wards.

The theoretical distribution of the chi-square statistic is a family of curves (like t-distributions) varying slightly in shape according to the degrees of freedom associated with the test. The degrees of freedom associated with a chi-square goodness of fit test are *one less* than the number of categories in the model. The χ^2 test is a non-directional test, and since each difference adds to the χ^2 statistic, the critical region for rejection always lies under the right-hand tail of the χ^2 distribution. Tables are available which list critical values of the statistic for each curve and common significance levels. Figure 13.2 shows how χ^2 distributions vary according to the degrees of freedom being used.

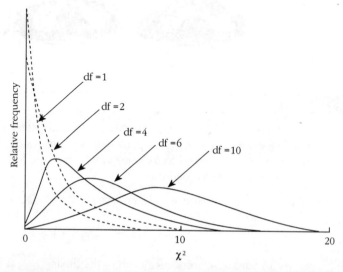

Figure 13.2 The variation in χ^2 distributions according to the degrees of freedom being used.(*Source* Pagano, R 1986, *Understanding Statistics in Behavioral Sciences*, 2nd edn, West Publishing Company, St Paul, Minnesota)

EXAMPLE **13.2**

In 1986 the proportions of people working in health and health-related occupations were: 59.1% in hospitals and nursing homes, 11% in medicine, 2.5% in community health centres, 11.2% in areas such as dental, optometry and ambulance, and 16.2% in other areas not stated.

A recent survey of 770 health workers yielded the following results:

Hospitals and nursing homes	509
Medicine	85
Community health centres	55
Dental, optometry and ambulance	97
Other areas not stated	24

Do these results suggest that the composition of people working in these areas has changed since the 1986 data was collected? Test at the 5% level of significance.

Solution

H_0: The proportions remain the same.
H_1: The proportions have altered.

With $5 - 1 = 4$ degrees of freedom critical $\chi^2 = 9.488$ at $\alpha = 0.05$

To calculate the expected frequencies we proceed as follows:

	O	E
Hospitals and nursing homes	509	59.1% of 770 = 455.07
Medicine	85	11.0% of 770 = 84.7
Community health centres	55	2.5% of 770 = 19.25
Dental, optometry and ambulance	97	11.2% of 770 = 86.24
Other areas not stated	24	16.2% of 770 = 124.74

$$\chi^2 = \sum \frac{(O - E)^2}{E}$$

$$= \frac{(509 - 455.07)^2}{455.07} + \frac{(85 - 84.7)^2}{84.7} + \frac{(55 - 19.25)^2}{19.25} + \frac{(97 - 86.24)^2}{86.24} + \frac{(24 - 124.74)^2}{124.74}$$

$$= 6.391 + 0.001 + 66.393 + 1.343 + 81.358 = 155.49$$

As the obtained value of 155.49 lies beyond the critical value of 9.488 there is overwhelming evidence that the composition of health workers has indeed changed. The most significant changes appear to have been in the areas of community health centres (a higher proportion than expected) and in other areas not stated where there has been a considerable decline.

13.2   Chi-square test of independence (two variables)

Another chi-square test that is very common in many areas of research involves data that are presented in the form of a contingency table. In this case we are dealing with more than one variable and are therefore most interested in whether or not one variable is influencing the other. For example, does music preference depend upon age? Are certain occupations biased towards males or females? Do people working in health occupations choose to do so because their parents have also worked in these areas?

A chi-square test may be used to establish whether two categorical variables are dependent or independent. For example, is the cause of death for children aged under 1 year associated with the sex of the child? This question is explored in Example 13.3.

EXAMPLE **13.3**

A study was undertaken for a sample of 90 male and 72 female deaths of children aged under 1 year. The results are tabulated below.

Cause of death	Males	Females	Total
Perinatal conditions	39	29	68
Congenital anomalies	21	19	40
All other causes	30	24	54
Total	90	72	162

Is there evidence to suggest that cause of death and sex of the child are related?

Solution

H_0: Cause of death is independent of gender.

H_1: Proportions for causes differ between males and females.

To calculate the expected frequencies for the table, we proceed as follows, assuming the null hypothesis to be true:

Since $\frac{90}{162}$ (55.6%) of total deaths were males then we should expect 55.6% of the 68 perinatal deaths to be male, $\frac{90}{162}$ of the 40 congenital deaths to be male and 55.6% of the remaining 54 deaths from all other causes to be male. Similarly, the proportion of female deaths should be $\frac{72}{162}$ (44.4%) of the deaths in each category. The table below includes the observed values plus the expected values calculated as outlined above. The expected values are in brackets.

Cause of death	Males	Females	Total
Perinatal conditions	39 (37.8)	29 (30.2)	68
Congenital anomalies	21 (22.2)	19 (17.8)	40
All other causes	30 (30)	24 (24)	54
Total	90	72	162

Now we can calculate the χ^2 statistic as usual:

$$\chi^2 = \sum \frac{(O-E)^2}{E} = 0.038 + 0.048 + 0.065 + 0.081 + 0 + 0 = 0.232$$

With two degrees of freedom and $\alpha = 0.05$, the critical value for χ^2 is 5.991. The obtained value for χ^2 is not beyond the critical value, so we fail to reject the null hypothesis and conclude that the cause of death is independent of sex.

The degrees of freedom for the above test is the product of the (number of rows − 1) and the (number of columns − 1), which in this case is (3 − 1)(2 − 1) = 2. What this means is that of the *six* cells in the body of the table only *two* need to be known in order to be able to calculate the remaining four. This assumes that the row totals and the column totals are given.

Using Minitab to perform a chi-square test

To make use of Minitab the data should be entered into columns, following the same pattern as the contingency table. Neither the row totals nor column totals are included. In this case the male deaths would be entered into column 1 and the female deaths into column 2. The appropriate command is CHISQUARE followed by the names of the columns into which the numerical data has been entered. Notice that the Minitab printout includes the expected values, and both row and column totals in addition to the degrees of freedom and the observed χ^2 value.

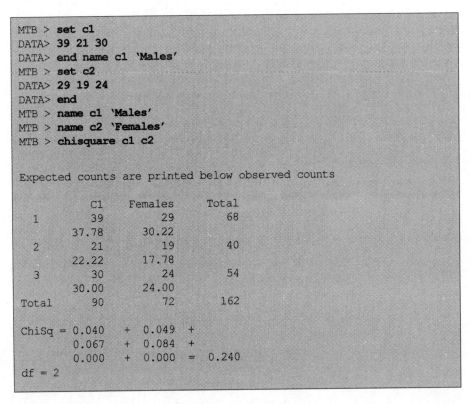

```
MTB > set c1
DATA> 39 21 30
DATA> end name c1 'Males'
MTB > set c2
DATA> 29 19 24
DATA> end
MTB > name c1 'Males'
MTB > name c2 'Females'
MTB > chisquare c1 c2


Expected counts are printed below observed counts

            C1     Females    Total
     1      39        29        68
          37.78     30.22
     2      21        19        40
          22.22     17.78
     3      30        24        54
          30.00     24.00
  Total     90        72       162


ChiSq = 0.040  +  0.049  +
        0.067  +  0.084  +
        0.000  +  0.000  =  0.240
  df = 2
```

Figure 13.3 Minitab printout for Example 13.3.

Chi-square tests are very common because they are used for categorical data. They are *not* used to test a hypothesis regarding some population parameter, so therefore do not involve sample means, standard deviations, confidence intervals, and the like. However, there are some limitations to the use of these tests that you should be aware of:

(a) Expected frequencies must not be too small. No expected frequency should be less than 1, and not more than 20% of the cells should have expected frequencies less than 5. This is not a problem if the sample size is sufficiently large. If this situation does occur it can be overcome by *merging* some of the rows or the columns so that the frequencies of the resulting cells increase to more acceptable levels.

(b) The obtained data must represent independent observations. For example, a person should not be included more than once when an experiment involves before *and* after observations, or when multiple responses are recorded for the same person.

(c) For 2 × 2 contingency tables the degrees of freedom is only equal to *one* and the approximation of the theoretical chi-square distribution to the discrete sampling distribution is not as good. This is offset to a large degree if the expected cell frequencies are large (ie greater than 10).

1   A health worker wishes to investigate whether the incidence of mumps varies throughout the year, or whether it remains constant. For the 96 cases of mumps recorded in the previous year the distribution was as follows:

J	F	M	A	M	J	J	A	S	O	N	D
2	6	4	4	8	10	8	6	6	10	10	6

What can be concluded on the basis of the above data? Test at the 5% level.

2   The police keep data on arrests for violent crimes according to the type of crime committed and the age of the person arrested. To test whether there is an association between these two characteristics, 750 arrest records for violent crimes are randomly selected. The sample results are displayed in the table below.

	18–24	25–44	45+
Murder	11	16	4
Rape	21	26	4
Robbery	128	92	6
Assault	162	234	46

(a) Calculate the row and column totals.

(b) Is there evidence that an association exists between the type of violent crime committed and the age of the person arrested? Use $\alpha = 0.01$.

3   A gambler thinks that a die may be 'loaded'; that is, he thinks that the probabilities for the six numbers may not be equal. To test his theory he rolls the die 150 times and obtains the following results:

Number	Frequency
1	23
2	26
3	23
4	21
5	31
6	26

(a) How many sixes would you expect to throw?

(b) Do the overall results indicate that the die is loaded? Use $\alpha = 0.05$.

4   It has been suggested that mature-age students perform better in first-year nursing courses than students who have come straight from secondary school. In an attempt to test this hypothesis, results from various universities were collected and considered in the light of the time that had elapsed since a student had finished school and commenced study. This is summarised in the table below.

Grade	Time elapsed (years)			
	0	1–4	5–10	>10
A	43	28	19	25
B	126	64	24	32
C	175	73	21	28
D	214	81	23	31
E	162	52	16	21
F	73	42	9	7

Is there evidence to support the above theory at the 5% level of significance?

5   Many insurance companies question the policy of offering reduced rates for small cars, since the companies claim that the rate of serious and fatal accidents is higher for those cars than for larger cars. To investigate this issue, an analysis of accident data was made to determine the distribution of numbers of cases in which at least one individual was fatally or critically injured for vehicles of three sizes. The data for 346 accidents are shown in the table. Do these data indicate that the frequency of fatal and critical injuries in auto accidents depends on the size of the car?

Injury	Small	Medium	Large
Fatal/critical	67	26	16
Not fatal or critical	128	63	46

6   A machine is supposed to mix dried sultanas, apricots, prunes and apples in the weight-ratio 5:2:2:1. A packet containing 500 g of these mixed dried fruits was found to have 269 g sultanas, 112 g apricots, 74 g prunes and 45 g apples. At the 5% level of significance, test the hypothesis that the machine is mixing the fruits in the correct ratio.

7   The grades in a nursing course for a particular semester were as follows:

Grade	A	B	C	D	E
Frequency	14	18	32	20	16

Test the hypothesis that the distribution of grades is uniform. Use $\alpha = 0.05$.

8 In an experiment to study the dependence of hypertension on smoking habits, the following data were collected for 180 individuals:

Condition	Non-smokers	Moderate	Heavy
Hypertension	21	36	30
No hypertension	48	26	19

Test the hypothesis that the presence or absence of hypertension is independent of smoking habits. Use a 5% level of significance.

9 A random sample of 90 adults is classified according to sex and the number of hours spent watching television during a week.

TV hours	Male	Female
≥ 25	15	29
< 25	27	19

Use a 0.01 level of significance and test the hypothesis that the time spent watching television is independent of whether the viewer is male or female.

10 A random sample of mothers were classified according to education and the number of children they had had:

Education	0–1 children	2–3 children	>3 children
Primary	14	37	32
Secondary	19	42	17
Tertiary	12	17	10

Test the hypothesis (at $\alpha = 0.05$) that the size of the family is independent of the level of education attained by the mother.

11 Three cards are drawn from an ordinary deck of playing cards, with replacement, and the number of spades is recorded. After repeating the experiment 64 times the following table resulted:

No. of spades	0	1	2	3
Frequency	21	31	12	0

Test the hypothesis that the recorded data may be fitted by the binomial distribution where $n = 3$ and $p = 0.25$.

12 The following survival data was collected on 100 widows and 100 widowers following the death of a spouse:

Years lived	Widow	Widower
Less than 5	25	39
5 to 10	42	40
More than 10	33	21

Can we conclude at the 0.05 level of significance that the proportions of widows and widowers are equal with respect to the different time periods that they survive after the death of their spouse?

13 In a study to estimate the proportion of people who regularly watch live television shows, it is found that 52 of 200 people in Melbourne, 31 of 150 people in Sydney and 37 of 150 people in Canberra watch at least one live television show. Use $\alpha = 0.05$ to test the hypothesis that there is no difference among the true proportions of people who watch live television shows in these three cities.

14 The table below gives the distribution of the marital status of persons aged 15 years or more in Australia at the time of the 1986 Census.

Marital status	Relative frequency
Never Married	0.284
Married	0.578
Separated (not divorced)	0.026
Divorced	0.047
Widowed	0.065

By means of comparison, a random sample of 500 Ballarat residents aged 15 years and over yielded the following results:

Marital status	Frequency
Never Married	100
Married	250
Separated (not divorced)	42
Divorced	58
Widowed	50

Is there evidence to suggest that the marital status distribution in Ballarat differs from that of the nation as a whole?

CHAPTER OUTLINE

CHAPTER FOURTEEN

One-way analysis of variance

LEARNING OBJECTIVES

After reading this chapter you should be able to:
- discuss what is being measured with the between-groups variance estimate and the within-groups variance estimate;
- evaluate a ratio of variances and compare this with critical values in tables for the F distribution;
- write suitable hypotheses for the comparison of the means of several groups;
- calculate the within-groups variance estimate;
- calculate the between-groups variance estimate;
- calculate the degrees of freedom associated with each estimate;
- complete an ANOVA table; and
- use and interpret the output which results from the Minitab commands AOVO and ONEWAY.

In previous chapters we looked at methods for comparing the means or medians of two independent populations. These methods made use of hypothesis tests such as independent *t*-tests, *z*-tests and Mann–Whitney tests. In each case we restricted ourselves to two samples. Now we shall consider how means from more than two samples can be compared. For example, we might wish to determine which of several treatments for a disease is the best, or which of several brands of running shoe absorbs shock to the greatest degree, or whether or not different levels of experience have any influence over worker efficiency. Many such situations involving differences among several samples occur in research problems, so we need a procedure to deal with the problem of comparing means from more than two populations. The procedure that has been developed for this purpose is referred to as *analysis of variance* (*ANOVA*). The testing procedure that we use is referred to as an *F-test*.

14.1 Rationale for analysis of variance

It may seem odd that a test comparing several population means is called an 'analysis of variance'! Figures 14.1 and 14.2 may help to explain. Figure 14.1 shows three possible samples taken from three populations having the same shape but different means. This is an important point, because if the populations have the same shape then this implies that they have the same variance. The only way they can differ is if they have different means. The second diagram shows the three samples *combined* as though they have been taken from a common population with a large variance. The following question naturally arises: Is the variation that we observe in the scores due to the large variance of a common population (Figure 14.2), or is it due to actual differences in the sample means (Figure 14.1)?

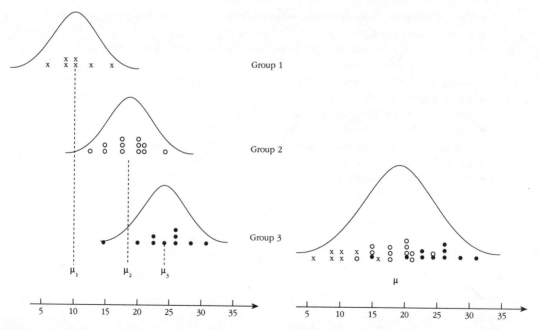

Figure 14.1 Three apparently different populations.

Figure 14.2 A conceivable common population

If the observed variation is due simply to a large variation in a common population, then by estimating this common variance in two ways we can determine an answer to the question. The more similar the two variance estimates are, the more likely the scores have come from a common population. It is in this way that we can determine whether or not there are differences between sample means.

14.2 The F-test

The *F*-test is named after R.A. Fisher, who was a pioneer in the field of experimental design; it involves calculating two estimates of a population variance. (We have already used this test in Section 11.3 when dealing with two samples.) The two estimates are expressed as a ratio, which is called the *F*-statistic. The *F*-statistic is therefore a measure of the *difference* between the two variance estimates calculated. If these variance estimates are similar, then the *F*-statistic will be close to 1. On the other hand, if the variance estimates are quite different then the F-statistic will be much larger, or much smaller than 1. What constitutes 'much larger' or 'much smaller' or 'close to' depends upon the level of significance chosen for the test.

Before going any further we should consider the assumptions under which the ANOVA test is carried out:

1   We assume that the populations from which the samples were taken are normally distributed;

2   We assume that the samples are both independent and randomly chosen; and

3   We assume that the samples have been drawn from populations having equal variances.

The first two assumptions are the same as those encountered previously when using *t*-tests and *z*-tests. The final assumption of equal variances has also been met before when using the *t*-test for independent groups with a pooled estimate of the variance. In the case of the *t*-test equal population variances are not assumed; rather their occurrence gives rise to a specific technique. On the other hand, we cannot perform an analysis of variance without assuming that the population variances are equal. We make this assumption because we only want the populations to differ by location (ie means). This is shown in Figure 14.1, in which the three different populations have the same variance but different means.

The null hypothesis assumes that there is no difference among the sample means; that is, all the sample means are equal. We state this accordingly:

$$H_0: \quad \mu_1 = \mu_2 = \mu_3 = \ldots = \mu_k$$

Note that μ_i represents the mean of the *i*th sample. The implication of this is that the scores in each sample have been randomly chosen from populations having the same mean value, which implies that the samples have actually come from a common population. If not enough evidence can be found to reject the null hypothesis, we conclude that the samples have come from a common population. In other words, there is no significant difference between any of the sample means.

The alternative hypothesis is non-directional and states that the means are not all the same. That is, that one or more of the sample means is significantly different from at least one of the others. This can be expressed as

$$H_1: \quad \mu_i \neq \mu_j \text{ for some } i, j$$

By making the three initial assumptions we are saying that the populations have the same shape. The only way left for them to differ is in terms of their location. We know that ANOVA involves calculating two variance estimates and expressing them as a ratio, but the way in which an analysis of variance actually tests for differences between several means can be seen by the manner in which the variance estimates are determined.

14.3 Estimating a common population variance

One way to estimate a population variance is to average the sample variances. We call this the *within-groups estimate of variance*, since each sample variance reflects only the variation within a particular group. This estimate is designated by the term s_w^2.

A second estimate of a population variance can be found indirectly from the Central Limit Theorem using the result $\sigma_{\bar{x}}^2 = \frac{\sigma^2}{n}$. We have a set of sample means that, if H_0 is true, have all come from the same sampling distribution. Finding the variance of these sample means will enable us to estimate the population variance. We refer to this as the *between-groups estimate of the variance* and denote it by the term s_b^2.

The *F*-statistic is then defined as the ratio of these two estimates:

$$F = \frac{s_b^2}{s_w^2}$$

14.4 Calculating the variance estimates

In estimating a common population variance we have assumed that all the samples have been taken from populations having equal variances. That is,

$$\sigma_1^2 = \sigma_2^2 = \sigma_3^2 = ... = \sigma_k^2$$

We know that each sample variance is an unbiased estimate of the population variance, σ^2. By pooling the sample variances, ie averaging them, we can obtain an even better estimate for σ^2, expressed as follows:

$$s_w^2 = \frac{s_1^2 + s_2^2 + s_3^2 + ... + s_k^2}{k}$$

If the sample sizes are not the same then the sample variances are *weighted* according to their respective degrees of freedom. This means that we divide by the *total* number of observations *less* the number of samples used. Hence we would have

$$s_w^2 = \frac{(n_1 - 1)s_1^2 + (n_2 - 1)s_2^2 + (n_3 - 1)s_3^2 + ... + (n_k - 1)s_k^2}{(n_1 + n_2 + n_3 + ... n_k) - k}$$

where n_1 represents the size of sample 1, etc. and there are k samples altogether. This estimate of the common population variance for the samples does not depend upon the truth or falsity of the null hypothesis, since s is calculated on each sample separately. This is why we use this particular estimate in the denominator of the definition for F.

The second variance estimate, s_b^2, is based upon the means of the samples. According to the null hypothesis these sample means are all equal, and if this is true we can say that these means have been drawn from the same population. Therefore we can use the variance of the sample means to obtain an estimate for σ^2. This can be obtained indirectly from the Central Limit Theorem as follows:

The variance of sample means is given by

$$\sigma_{\bar{x}}^2 = \frac{\sigma_x^2}{n}$$

which implies that

$$\sigma_x^2 = n.\sigma_{\bar{x}}^2$$

This forms the basis for the second estimate of the common population variance. As we are dealing with samples, we use $s_{\bar{x}}^2$ as an *unbiased* estimate of the variance of the treatment means. We have

$$s_b^2 = n.s_{\bar{x}}^2$$

where n refers to the size of each sample. This method obviously assumes that each sample is of the same size. Example 14.1 is an illustration of this conceptual approach to the analysis of variance.

EXAMPLE 14.1

Nursing staff at an American hospital were interested to see if there were significant differences in the weights of new-born babies according to the age of the mothers. Six births were randomly chosen from each of four age groupings and the weights of the babies at birth were noted (in lbs). The results appear below:

Mother's age (years)			
<20	20<25	25<30	30+
6.5	6	8.5	7
5	7.5	7	6.5
3.5	8	7	7.5
4	5.5	4.5	8.5
3	6	6.5	6
4.5	9	7.5	5

Does the data provide significant evidence that weights of new-born babies are different for mothers of varying ages? Test at the 5% level of significance.

Solution

H_0: The means for each age group are the same.

H_1: The means for each age group are not all the same.

From the above data we have the following summary statistics:

Statistic	Mother's age (years)			
	<20	20<25	25<30	30+
Sample means	4.42	7.0	6.83	6.75
Sample variances	1.54	1.9	1.77	1.48

EXAMPLE **14.1**   **cont.**

1   Calculate the two estimates of the overall variance.

(a) The within-groups variance estimate (mean of the group variances).
$$s_w^2 = \frac{1.54 + 1.9 + 1.77 + 1.48}{4} = \frac{6.69}{4} = 1.67$$

(b) The between-groups variance estimate (using variance of group means).
$s_b^2 = n.s_{\bar{x}}^2$ where $n = 6$ and $s_{\bar{x}}^2$ = variance of group means = 1.50
$s_b^2 = 6(1.50) = 9$

2   Calculate the value of the test statistic.
$$F = \frac{s_b^2}{s_w^2} = \frac{9}{1.67} = 5.34$$

3   Compare the value obtained above with a critical F-value.
Since two estimates of variance are involved in the calculation of F, there are two values used for the degrees of freedom associated with the F-statistic. We have one value for the numerator, and one for the denominator. As there are k groups there are $(k-1)$ degrees of freedom associated with the numerator. The degrees of freedom for the denominator is given by $N - k$ where N represents the sum of the sample sizes ie N = total number of observations. Note that the total degrees of freedom is $(k-1) + (N-k) = N-1$. In this example we have four groups and 24 values, therefore we have three degrees of freedom for the numerator and 20 degrees of freedom for the denominator. Thus the critical F-value is $F_{3,20} = 3.10$ using the required α-level of 5%.

4   Conclusion
As the obtained F-value of 5.34 is beyond the critical F-value of 3.10, we reject H_0 and conclude that at least one of the sample means is different.

While the method in Example 14.1 conceptually demonstrates what happens in an analysis of variance, the usual method for ANOVA involves the calculation of what we call *sums of squares*. The sums of squares are defined as the numerators of the two variance estimates used in Example 14.1.

14.5   ANOVA using sums of squares

Using the sums of squares approach is more accurate than the conceptual method because it involves dealing with the *raw scores* rather than the summary statistics. Summary statistics such as the mean and the standard deviation are often rounded, and repeated use of them in formulae can lead to a build-up of error. Also, the sums of squares method does not require each group to have equal sample sizes, and is therefore more widely usable.

The total sum of squares (SS_T) is defined in the usual manner as the sum of the squared deviations of each score from the mean. The mean in this instance refers to the *overall mean* (the mean of all of the scores combined). SS_T is found as follows:

$$SS_T = \Sigma X^2 - \frac{(\Sigma X)^2}{N}$$

where N = total number of observations.

The total sum of squares can be broken up into two components — sums of squares *within the groups* (SS_W) and sums of squares *between the groups* (SS_B). These two components of the total sum of squares are defined as follows:

$$SS_W = \sum X^2 - \left(\frac{T_1^2}{n_1} + \frac{T_2^2}{n_2} + \frac{T_3^2}{n_3} + \ldots + \frac{T_k^2}{n_k} \right)$$

where T_1^2 = sum of the scores (ie total) from the ith group squared, and
$\quad n_i$ = the number of scores in the ith group.

$$SS_B = \left(\frac{T_1^2}{n_1} + \frac{T_2^2}{n_2} + \frac{T_3^2}{n_3} + \ldots + \frac{T_k^2}{n_k} \right) - \frac{(\sum X)^2}{N}$$

By combining the within-groups sum of squares and the between-groups sum of squares, we get the total sum of squares. That is,

$$SS_T = SS_W + SS_B$$

In practice we need only to calculate two of the above sums of squares given the relationship immediately above. Usually we calculate SS_T and SS_B, and then obtain SS_W by subtraction. After the respective sums of squares have been calculated, the results are summarised in the form of a table. The variance estimates s_b^2 and s_w^2, traditionally called *mean squares*, are each determined by dividing the appropriate sums of squares by the respective degrees of freedom. The F-ratio is found by dividing the between-groups variance estimate by the within-groups variance estimate.

Table 14.1 Summary table for ANOVA calculations.

Source of variation	Degrees of freedom	Sums of squares	Variance estimates	F-ratio
Between groups	$k-1$	SS_B	s_b^2	$\dfrac{s_b^2}{s_w^2}$
Within groups	$N-k$	SS_W	s_w^2	
Total	$N-1$	SS_T		

Example 14.2 demonstrates the use of the sums of squares approach with the same data used in Example 14.1. The results will be placed into an ANOVA summary table. The slight differences from Example 14.1 occur because of the rounding errors associated with using sample means and sample standard deviations rather than raw scores.

EXAMPLE **14.2**

Nursing staff at an American hospital were interested to see if there were significant differences in the weights of new-born babies according to the age of the mothers. Six births were randomly chosen from each of four age-groupings and the weights of the babies at birth were noted (in lbs). The results appear on the following page:

EXAMPLE 14.2

cont.

	Mother's age (years)		
<20	20 < 25	25 < 30	30+
6.5	6	8.5	7
5	7.5	7	6.5
3.5	8	7	7.5
4	5.5	4.5	8.5
3	6	6.5	6
4.5	9	7.5	5
26.5	42	41	40.5

Does the data provide significant evidence that weights of new-born babies are different for mothers of varying ages? Test at the 5% level of significance.

Solution

H_0: The means for each age group are the same.

H_1: The means for each age group are not all the same

From the above data we also have:

$\sum X = 150$, $\sum X^2 = 998$, $N = 24$, $k = 4$ groups.

1 Calculation of sums of squares.

$$SS_T = \sum X^2 - \frac{(\sum X^2)}{N} = 998 - \frac{(150)^2}{N} = 998 - 937.5 = 60.5$$

$$SS_B = \sum \frac{T^2}{n} - \frac{(\sum X)^2}{N} = \left(\frac{(26.5)^2}{6} + \frac{(42)^2}{6} + \frac{(41)^2}{6} + \frac{(40.5)^2}{6} \right) - 937.5$$

$$SS_B = 964.58 - 937.5 = 27.08$$

$$SS_W = SS_T - SS_B = 60.5 - 27.08 = 33.42$$

2 Summarise the results in the form of an ANOVA table.

Source	d.f.	SS	s^2	F
Between groups	3	27.08	9.03	5.40
Within groups	20	33.42	1.67	
Total	23	60.50		

3 State a conclusion, using $\alpha = 0.05$ and critical $F_{3,20} = 3.10$.

The obtained $F = 5.40$ is beyond the critical $F = 3.10$, so we can reject H_0 and conclude that at least one of the sample means is significantly different. From the data it would appear that mothers less than 20 years of age had babies that were significantly lighter than those from other age groups.

14.6 ANOVA using Minitab

Example 14.2 demonstrates the considerable amount of calculation that is involved in performing an analysis of variance test. Fortunately we have access to computer packages today that enable us to perform these arduous calculations quite easily. Minitab will perform an analysis of variance as long as the data for each group is put into separate columns. The printout below was obtained for the data used in Examples 14.1 and 14.2. Notice how the data for mothers aged less than 20 years has been entered into column 1, the data for mothers aged from 20 < 25 years has been entered into column 2, etc. There are two Minitab commands that can be used for analysis of variance. The first is AOVO (Analysis Of Variance, Oneway) which requires the columns to be stipulated, as shown in Figure 14.3. The second command is ONEWAY, which requires all of the data to be in one column with codes for treatment groups in a second column (Figure 14.4).

```
MTB > print c1-c4

 ROW   <20Yrs   20<25   25<30   30+Yrs

   1     6.5      6.0     8.5     7.0
   2     5.0      7.5     7.0     6.5
   3     3.5      8.0     7.0     7.5
   4     4.0      5.5     4.5     8.5
   5     3.0      6.0     6.5     6.0
   6     4.5      9.0     7.5     5.0


MTB > aovo c1-c4

ANALYSIS OF VARIANCE
SOURCE    DF      SS       MS       F       P
FACTOR     3    27.08     9.03    5.40    0.007
ERROR     20    33.42     1.67
TOTAL     23    60.50
                             INDIVIDUAL 95 PCT CI'S FOR MEAN
                             BASED ON POOLED STDEV
 LEVEL     N    MEAN    STDEV  --------+---------+---------+---------
 <20Yrs    6   4.417   1.242  (-------*-------)
 20<25     6   7.000   1.378                 (--------*------)
 25<30     6   6.833   1.329                (-------*------)
 30+Yrs    6   6.750   1.214                (------*------)
                              --------+---------+---------+---------
 POOLED STDEV =   1.293           4.5       6.0       7.5
```

Figure 14.3 Minitab printout of the ANOVA for Example 14.2 using the AOVO command.

The summary table produced by Minitab also includes the p-value, which can be directly compared to the chosen α-level. If the p-value is greater than the α-level, H_0 is accepted. The printout also contains a set of confidence intervals (95%) for the means of each of the groups. These confidence intervals are based upon a *pooled* standard deviation rather than the *individual* standard deviations of each of the groups, but they do provide a good visual indication of the groups that are likely to be significantly different. Notice also that the Minitab printout uses the terms 'factor' and 'error' to describe the sources of variation, rather than 'between groups' and 'within groups'. The column containing the estimates for the variance is headed MS, which stands for mean sum of squares.

14.7   Summary

ANOVA is a statistical technique for analysing multigroup experiments, usually with more than two groups or treatments. The F-test allows us to make one overall comparison which determines whether there is a significant difference between the means of the groups. Making only one comparison avoids the problem of an increased Type I error which would occur if group means were compared two at a time using the t-test for independent groups.

To test H_0 we calculate two estimates of the population variance. One of these, the within-groups variance estimate, s_w^2, is independent of the truth or falsity of the null hypothesis. The second estimate of the population variance is called the between-groups variance estimate, s_b^2, which does depend upon the null hypothesis. If both estimates are similar we have no reason to reject H_0. However, if the two estimates disagree we conclude that underlying differences in the treatment means have contributed to the between-groups estimate, inflating it and causing it to differ from the first. We therefore reject the null hypothesis.

A final example shows the sums of squares approach for samples of unequal size. Note the effect of unequal sample sizes in the calculation of SS_w.

EXAMPLE 14.3

Patients suffering from a particular stomach ailment were given three different sorts of treatment, and their recovery rates were monitored. The results are tabulated below. Use a 5% level of significance to decide whether there is a difference in recovery rates for the different treatments.

Treatment	Days to recovery
A	6, 9, 7, 3, 8, 4
B	7, 6, 9, 5, 5, 6, 5
C	4, 3, 5, 2, 6

Solution

H_0:   The means for each treatment group are the same.
H_1:   The means for each treatment group are not all the same.

From the data we also have:

$T_A = 37$, $T_B = 43$, $T_C = 20$, $\Sigma X = 100$, $\Sigma X^2 = 622$, $N = 18$, $k = 3$, $n_A = 6$, $n_B = 7$, $n_C = 5$.

1   Calculate sums of squares.

$$SS_T = \Sigma X^2 - \frac{(\Sigma X)^2}{N} = 662 - \frac{(100)^2}{18} = 622 - 555.56 = 66.44$$

$$SS_B = \Sigma \frac{T^2}{n_1} - \frac{(\Sigma X)^2}{N} = \left(\frac{(37)^2}{6} + \frac{(43)^2}{7} + \frac{(20)^2}{5} \right) - 555.56$$

$$SS_B = 572.31 - 555.56 = 16.75$$

$$SS_W = SS_T - SS_B = 66.44 - 16.75 = 49.69$$

2   Summarise the results in the form of an ANOVA table.

Source	d.f.	SS	s^2	F
Between groups	2	16.75	8.38	2.53
Within groups	15	49.69	3.31	
Total	17	66.44		

3   State a conclusion, using $\alpha = 0.05$ and critical $F_{2,15} = 3.68$.

The obtained $F = 2.53$ is not beyond the critical $F = 3.68$, so we cannot reject H_0. We conclude that there is no significant difference between the sample means and therefore no difference in the recovery rates for each of the treatments.

Figure 14.4 is the Minitab printout of the analysis for Example 14.3 using the ONEWAY command. The data for all three treatments was entered into column 1, with the following codes entered into column 2:

    0 = Treatment A, 1 = Treatment B, 2 = Treatment C

```
MTB > set c1
DATA> 6 9 7 3 8 4 7 6 9 5 5 6 5 4 3 5 2 6
DATA> end
MTB > set c2
DATA> 6(0) 7(1) 5(2)
DATA> end
MTB name c2 'treatment'
MTB > oneway c1 c2


ANALYSIS OF VARIANCE ON C1
SOURCE    DF      SS      MS      F       p
C2        2     16.75    8.38   2.53   0.113
ERROR    15     49.69    3.31
TOTAL    17     66.44
                        INDIVIDUAL 95 PCT CI'S FOR MEAN
                        BASED ON POOLED STDEV
LEVEL    N     MEAN    STDEV -----+---------+---------+---------+-
    0    6    6.167    2.317                 (---------*---------)
    1    7    6.143    1.464                 (---------*--------)
    2    5    4.000    1.581   (------------*-----------)
                            -----+---------+---------+---------+-
POOLED STDEV =  1.820        3.0      4.5      6.0      7.5
```

Figure 14.4 Minitab printout of the ANOVA for Example 14.3 using the ONEWAY command.

The diagram of the 95% confidence intervals for the means shows that the mean recovery time for treatment C (coded as 2) appears to be less than the other two treatments. This has been highlighted in italic type in the printout. This difference however is not significant at the 5% level, as indicated by the p-value of 0.113. To be significant at the 5% level the p-value needs to be <0.05. In fact a p-value of 0.113 indicates that the difference is not significant unless a significance level of 11.3% is used.

1 Consider an F-curve with df = (24,5).
   (a) How many degrees of freedom are associated with the numerator?
   (b) How many degrees of freedom are associated with the denominator?
   (c) Find the F-value with an area of 0.01 to its right.
   (d) Determine F for $\alpha = 0.05$.

2 Which two statistics are measures of variation between the sample means in a one-way ANOVA?

3 Which two statistics are measures of the variation within samples in one-way ANOVA?

4 Independent random samples of robbery reports from private homes, service stations and convenience stores have been collected and analysed with respect to the amounts of money stolen. The results are provided in the table below, with amounts given to the nearest dollar.

Private home	Service station	Convenience store
411	314	575
320	356	442
496	379	458
410	424	475
429	365	376
	532	548

   (a) Compute the sample means and the standard deviations for each of the three robbery groups.
   (b) Determine s_B^2 and s_W^2.
   (c) What do each of the terms in part (b) actually measure?
   (d) In order to carry out an analysis of variance what are we comparing, and what assumptions are necessary?

5 For a one-way ANOVA,
   (a) list and interpret the three sums of squares, and
   (b) state the assumptions which should be checked before using a one-way ANOVA.

6 A company wishes to test the market effect of four different designs for the container of one of its most unsuccessful products. The number of cases sold at each of five randomly selected outlets is recorded for each design. The results appear below. Does the data provide evidence of a difference in mean sales among the four designs at the 1% level?

Design A	Design B	Design C	Design D
41	51	44	58
51	65	58	37
52	35	37	24
50	66	75	54
43	57	54	65

7 The following data represent the final marks obtained by four groups of nursing students randomly chosen from classes in the following subjects: Nursing History, Nursing Practice, Biology, Mathematics.

History	Prac.	Biology	Maths
57	73	61	68
94	91	86	83
81	63	59	72
73	77	66	55
68	75	87	92

Use a 0.05 level of significance to test the hypothesis that the courses are of equal difficulty.

8 It has often been suggested that the weather can affect the moods of patients. A random sample of patients was selected and assigned at random to one of three groups. Each group was given a mood questionnaire. One group was tested on a day that was cold and rainy, a second was tested during a violent storm, and a third was tested on a bright, calm, sunny day.

Cold/wet 6, 9, 10, 12, 5, 7, 12, 8, 7, 10
Stormy   8, 6, 12, 10, 8, 9, 14, 7, 7, 10
Sunny   6, 8, 13, 10, 13, 10, 9, 12, 15, 11

Does it appear that the weather has an effect on the mood of patients? Use $\alpha = 0.05$.

9 The following summary table presents the results of an ANOVA from an experiment comparing four treatment conditions with a sample of $n = 10$ for each treatment. Complete the table and state a suitable conclusion.

Source	df	SS	MS	
Factor				F=8.00
Error		72		
Total				

Progress review 5

PART A Choose the correct answer for the following multiple-choice questions.

1 Which of the following is an example of an alternative hypothesis?
   (a) $\mu_1 = \mu_2$,
   (b) $\mu_1 - \mu_2 = 0$,
   (c) both of the above,
   (d) $\mu_1 < \mu_2$, or
   (e) none of the above.

2 Suppose samples were drawn from two populations that had different means. On the basis of the difference between the two sample means, the experimenter accepted H_1. Which answer describes this situation?
   (a) Type I error,
   (b) Type II error,
   (c) correct decision, or
   (d) either (a) or (b) depending on whether a one-tailed or two-tailed test was used.

3 What rank would a score of 4 have on the following distribution?
   1   22   3   4   4   4   5
   (a) 4,
   (b) 5.5,
   (c) 6,
   (d) 7, or
   (e) none of the above.

4 Non-parametric tests are used rather than a t-test or an ANOVA when
   (a) the researcher does not know the specific value of the population parameters,
   (b) the data are in the form of ranks,
   (c) the assumption of random sampling is not justified,
   (d) both (b) and (c), or
   (e) none of the above.

5 The non-parametric test that corresponds in design to the t-test for independent samples is the
   (a) Mann–Whitney test,
   (b) Wilcoxon signed-ranks test,
   (c) Sign test,
   (d) Chi-square test of independence, or
   (e) none of the above.

6 The null hypothesis for a goodness of fit test is that the observed frequencies
   (a) fit the expected frequencies,
   (b) do not fit the expected frequencies,
   (c) either of the above, depending on the size of the χ^2 value,
   (d) either of the above, depending on the degrees of freedom, or
   (e) are greater than the expected frequencies.

7 In a χ^2 test of independence between sex and kinds of phobias, H_0 was rejected.

The proper conclusion is that:

(a) sex and phobias are independent of each other,

(b) sex and phobias are related to each other,

(c) knowing a person's phobia gives you no clue to his or her sex,

(d) males have more phobias than females, or

(e) none of the above.

8 The null hypothesis tested by an ANOVA is that

(a) each sample is drawn from a different population,

(b) all samples have the same mean,

(c) the populations from which the samples are drawn have the same mean,

(d) at least one of the sample means is not the same as the others, or

(e) one or more of the populations from which the samples are drawn has a mean that is different from the others.

9 If H_0 is true, which of the following will be a good estimate of the population variance?

(a) mean square within groups,

(b) mean square between groups,

(c) both of the above, or

(d) none of the above.

PART B Write a short explanation (two to five lines) in answering each of the following questions.

10 Suppose 80 randomly selected residents are randomly divided into two groups. One group is given a glass of wine with dinner each evening for a month, and the other group is not. All subjects are then given a test of self-confidence in which higher scores mean greater self-confidence. The mean for the wine-with-dinner group is 77.3 and that for the non-wine group is 72.9. The z-score for this difference is 3.19. Write a suitable conclusion, including the p-value for this test.

11 When using Minitab to analyse the difference between means of independent samples, the experimenter can either use the POOLED subcommand or not. Explain this subcommand, why it should be used, when it should be used, and what it does.

12 An experimental automobile emission control system has been developed and the developers wish to find out if it will *decrease* fuel consumption. Eight cars are randomly selected. Each car is driven for 250 km using the standard emission system and then for 250 km using the experimental emission system. The same 8 drivers are used in each case. Fuel consumption is recorded and the results are listed below. Assuming the distribution of fuel consumption to be normal, does the data provide enough evidence to suggest that the experimental emission control system reduces fuel consumption? Test at the 5% level.

	Cars							
	1	2	3	4	5	6	7	8
Fuel consumption (litres) with standard emission control	17	23	27	14	28	21	29	13
Fuel consumption (litres) with experimental emission control	9	17	21	16	22	17	25	13

13 Use the most powerful non-parametric test that would be suitable to re-analyse the fuel consumption data above. Explain why you would use such a test.

14 A consumer protection agency wanted to test the hypothesis that the median cost of an automobile repair was the same in the metropolitan area as in nearby country centres. Estimates were obtained from metropolitan panel beaters as well as country panel beaters for a particular repair job. The estimates (in hundreds of dollars) were as follows:

Country	Metropolitan
77	68
80	71
85	73
90	92
92	97
	98
	98

Do the data provide sufficient evidence to indicate a difference in the median cost? Use a Mann–Whitney test with a 10% level of significance.

15 Assume that for tomatoes, the colour of the fruit and the height of the plant are genetically determined (with red dominant over yellow and tall dominant over short). A particular set of crossings will result in a 9 : 3 : 3 : 1 ratio (9 tall reds to 3 short reds to 3 tall yellows to 1 short yellow). Suppose you carried out the crossings and found 92 tall reds, 40 short reds, 39 tall yellows and 21 short yellows. Use an appropriate test to determine if such data fit a 9 : 3 : 3 : 1 model.

16 To test the hypothesis that style of leadership is likely to decrease absenteeism, an experiment was undertaken in a large city involving three hospitals. Twelve nurses were randomly assigned to one of the three hospitals. The three styles of leadership were: (1) Hospital A — bureaucratic; (2) Hospital B — paternalistic; (3) Hospital C — contractual.

The resulting absenteeism rates per employee after 6 months are presented in the Minitab printout.

(a) Test the null hypothesis that there is no difference in absenteeism among the different management styles.

(b) Use the printout to answer the following questions.

   (i) What is the value of the total sum of squares?

   (ii) What is the value of the between-groups estimate of the variance?

   (iii) At $\alpha = 5\%$, what is the critical F-value?

   (iv) Which style of leadership produced the highest level of absenteeism?

   (v) What is the probability of obtaining the result observed given that H_0 is true?

   (vi) Verify that the error mean square is equal to 0.858.

```
MTB > print c1-c3

ROW    Hos.A   Hos.B   Hos.C

 1      6.3     4.4     5.1
 2      7.1     5.2     5.5
 3      4.9     3.6     5.6
 4      6.8     5.4     3.5

MTB > aovo c1-c3
```

```
ANALYSIS OF VARIANCE
SOURCE    DF     SS      MS       F      p
FACTOR     2   6.052   3.026    3.53   .074
ERROR      9   7.725   0.858
TOTAL     11  13.777
                 INDIVIDUAL 95 PCT CI'S FOR MEAN
                 BASED ON POOLED STDEV
LEVEL      N    MEAN  STDEV ---------+---------+---------+---------
Hos.A      4  6.2750 0.9743                (---------*-------)
Hos.B      4  4.6500 0.8226 (-------*-------)
Hos.C      4  4.9250 0.9743   (-------*-------)
                             ---------+---------+---------+---------
POOLED STDEV = 0.9265                 4.8       6.0       7.2
```

Appendix 1
Decision flow charts

This Appendix consists of a series of decision flow charts which provide a summary of the basic statistical procedures covered in this text. These charts are meant to be read from left to right, and by following the relevant path, which will depend upon what you want to do and the nature of the data you have collected, you will be guided to the most appropriate procedure. The four charts include the following broad areas:

- descriptive statistics,
- hypothesis tests for means,
- non-parametric hypothesis tests, and
- measuring the relationship between two variables.

The charts do not cover every possibility, and need to be interpreted in the context of the material covered in this text. They are based upon similar charts developed by Gravetter and Wallnau (1992) in their text *Statistics for the Behavioural Sciences* (West Publishing, MN, USA).

Chart 1   Choosing appropriate descriptive statistics

The main purpose of descriptive statistics is to simplify and organise data by using tables or graphs, or by calculating appropriate summary statistics that describe certain attributes of the data. The scale of measurement that is used determines which of the procedures we adopt.

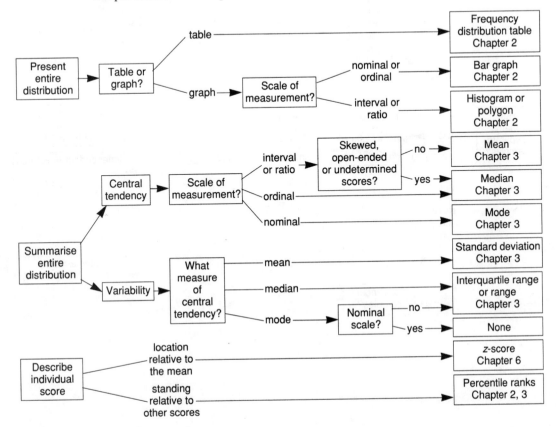

Chart 2   Choosing an appropriate hypothesis test for sample means

The hypothesis tests covered in this section are

- *single sample* hypothesis tests,
- two-sample hypothesis tests using *paired data* (data can be paired by using a repeated measures design where each subject is measured more than once, or by making a deliberate effort to match the subjects in some way), and
- two-sample hypothesis tests using *independent samples*.

All the tests in this section use sample means (or proportions) as the basis for testing hypotheses about the population parameters. Certain restrictions must be satisfied before these tests can be applied. These include:

- the use of an interval or ratio scale of measurement,
- the use of random sampling techniques, and
- appropriate conditions for the Central Limit Theorem to apply.

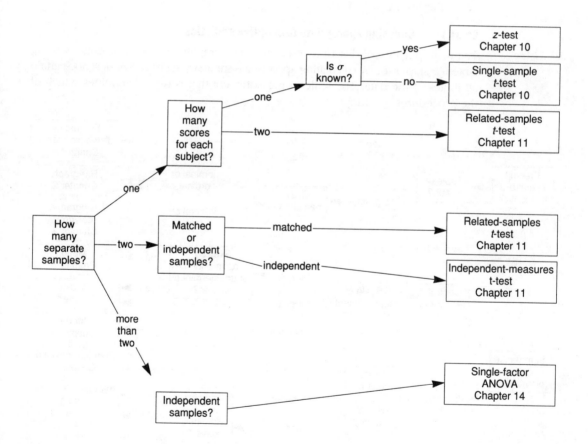

Chart 3   Choosing an appropriate non-parametric hypothesis test

Often a researcher finds that one or more of the conditions necessary for hypothesis tests such as those described above do not apply: distributions may be badly skewed or otherwise not normal, the data may involve nominal or ordinal scales of measurement, and so on. In these cases non-parametric hypothesis tests should be used. Generally they are quite straightforward as they do not involve the calculation of means or standard deviations.

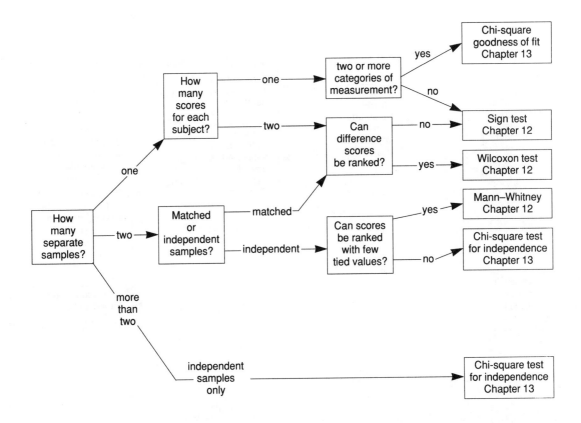

Chart 4   Measuring the relationship between two variables

Often it is important to know whether a relationship exists between two variables. Knowing the nature of such a relationship enables us to understand the behaviour of one variable given knowledge of the other. We may wish to predict values of one variable given particular values of another variable, or we might wish to determine the consistency or direction of the relationship. Different methods are used for specific types of data, so it is most important to determine the type of variable involved and the scale of measurement used to record the observations.

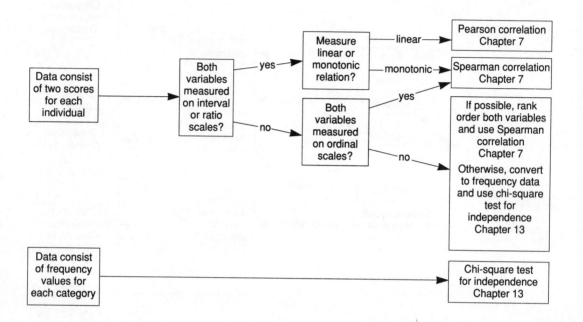

Appendix 2
Review of basic mathematical concepts

This Appendix reviews some of the basic mathematical concepts required for the statistical calculations used in this text. This review is meant to be used as a means of identifying where particular problems occur. Some students may need to do extensive work to bring their skills up to the level required, and may require assistance from a tutor. Do not be concerned if this is the case with you, because a thorough knowledge of this material now will make the rest of your statistics course much easier.

Before you proceed any further, check the table of symbols below. This table presents a summary of the mathematical symbols you should know.

Symbol	Meaning
$+, -, \times, \div$	Symbols representing *addition, subtraction, multiplication* and *division*; they are sometimes referred to as *operators*.
$<$	Symbol representing *less than*, eg $4 < 6$. Note that the small end points towards the smaller number.
$\leq$	This symbol means *less than or equal to*. For example, if $x \leq Y$ then the values represented by x are less than or equal to those represented by Y.
$>$	Symbol representing *greater than*, eg $6 > 4$.
$\geq$	This symbol means *greater than or equal to*.
$\neq$	Symbol meaning *not equal to*, eg $5 \neq 6$.
$\approx$	Symbol meaning *approximately equal to*, eg $\frac{1}{3} \approx 33\%$.
$\pm$	Symbol meaning *plus or minus*.
$\frac{1}{x}$	The *reciprocal* of x. This can be found on most calculators.
x^2	This is read as *x squared*, ie x multiplied by itself $x \times x$.
x^3	This is read as *x cubed*, or *x raised to the power of 3*. It means x multiplied by itself three times, ie $x^3 = x \times x \times x$
$\sqrt{x}$ or $x^{\frac{1}{2}}$	This is read as the *square root of x*. It means what number multiplied by itself gives the answer x. For example $\sqrt{16} = 4$ because $4 \times 4 = 16$.
Σ	This symbol is the Greek capital letter for S. In statistics we use this symbol to mean *sum of*. So Σx means *the sum of all of the x-values*. For example if x represents the even numbers between 1 and 10 then the *sum of x* is given by $\Sigma x = 2 + 4 + 6 + 8 + 10 = 30$

This review section begins with a self-assessment test. You should allow yourself about half an hour to complete as much of this test as you can. Make sure that you do the test in a suitable area — a place where you will not be interrupted. When you have finished the test you should correct it yourself using the answers provided at the end of this Appendix. If you get more than three questions wrong in any of the four parts of the test, you will most likely need some extra help in that area.

Self-assessment test

Answers are provided at the end of this Appendix

Part 1   Basic arithmetic

1 $5 + (-3) + (-2) + 4 =$

2 $8 - (-4) =$

3 $3 - 2 - (-5) =$

4 $4 + (-2) - 1 - (-6) - (-5) =$

5 $6 \times (-3) =$

6 $-4 \times (-3) =$

7 $-2 \times 9 =$

8 $-3 \times (-3) \times (-4) =$

9 $15 \div (-5) =$

10 $-21 \div (-3) =$

11 $-36 \div 9 =$

12 $-56 \div (-7) =$

TOTAL SCORE Part 1 ....

Part 2   Percentages and fractions

1 Express 40% as a fraction

2 The fraction $\frac{3}{5}$ corresponds to ....%

3 Convert $\frac{10}{16}$ to a decimal

4 $\frac{4}{7} + \frac{2}{7} =$

5 $3.625 + 0.275 =$

6 $\frac{2}{5} \times \frac{3}{4} =$

7 $\frac{3}{8} \times \frac{2}{3} =$

8 $4.6 \times 0.3 =$

9 $\frac{2}{5} \div \frac{3}{4} =$

10 $\frac{2.8}{0.4} =$

11 30% of a group of 60 students are nurses. How many of the group are nurses?

12 If four-fifths of students studying nursing are female, how many males would you expect in a group of 120 such students?

TOTAL SCORE Part 2 ....

Part 3   Solving equations

For each equation given below, find the missing value represented by x.

1 $x + 5 = 18$

2 $x - 12 = 4$

3 $16 = x - 7$

4 $4(x) = 24$

5 $64 = 8x$

6 $\dfrac{x}{6} = 4$

7 $12 = \dfrac{x}{3}$

8 $2x + 3 = 11$

9 $23 = 7x + 2$

10 $\dfrac{(x + 2)}{4} = 7$

11 $\dfrac{(x - 5)}{3} = 5$

12 $13 = 3x - 11$

TOTAL SCORE Part 3 ....

Part 4   Exponents and square roots

1 $5^2 =$

2 $\sqrt{36} =$

3 $4^2 + 3^3 =$

4 $(4 + 3)^2$

5 $\sqrt{25} - 16 =$

6 $\sqrt{25} + \sqrt{9} =$

7 $-2^5 =$

8 $-3^4 =$

9 $\sqrt{9} \times 5 =$

10 $\dfrac{36}{\sqrt{16}} =$

11 If $a = 2$ and $b = 4$, then $a^2 + b^2 =$

12 If $p = 3$ and $q = -2$, then $p^2 q^3 =$

TOTAL SCORE Part 4 ....

Review of basic arithmetic

Addition and subtraction

- The order in which you perform addition or subtraction is not important:
  For example, $3 + 4 - 2$ can be done by adding $3 + 4$ first, or by subtracting $4 - 2$ first. Either way the result is the same; ie $3 + 4 - 2 = 5$.
- To subtract a larger number from a smaller number, take the smaller from the larger and make the result *negative*.
  For example, $15 - 35 = -20$.
- When adding numbers that include negative values you can interpret the negative sign as subtraction.
  For example, $2 + (-3) + 5 = 2 - 3 + 5 = 4$.
- When subtracting negative numbers make them positive, and add.
  For example, $2 - (-3) + 5 = 2 + 3 + 5 = 10$.

Multiplication and division

- Numbers can be multiplied or divided in any order. For example,
  $2 \times 3 \times 4$ is the same as $3 \times 4 \times 2$ or $2 \times 4 \times 3$.
  Also, $6 \times 4 \div 2 \times 4 = 4 \div 2 \times 6$.
  The equations above may also be written as $\frac{6 \times 4}{2} = \frac{6}{2} \times 4$ or $6 \times \frac{4}{2}$
- Generally you should multiply or divide before you add or subtract.
  For example, $4 \times 2 + 6 \div 3 - 4 =$
  $$8 + 2 - 4 = 6$$
- Multiplication or division of numbers having the *same sign* (ie both +ve or both −ve) will result in a positive answer.
  For example, $4 \times 3 = 12$; $(-3)(-5) = 15$; $-10 \div -5 = 2$; $\frac{-10}{-5} = 2$.
- Multiplication or division of numbers having *different signs* (ie one +ve and one −ve) will result in a negative answer.
  For example, $-4 \times 3 = -12$; $3(-5) = -15$; $-10 \div 5 = -2$; $\frac{-10}{5} = -2$.
- Where brackets are involved in an expression perform the operations indicated inside the brackets before anything else.
  For example, $2 + 4(4 + 6 \div 2) = 2 + 4 \times 7 = 30$.

Review of fractions, decimals and percentages

What are fractions?

- Fractions consist of a *numerator* and a *denominator*. The *numerator* is the value on the top and the *denominator* is the value on the bottom.
  For example, the fraction two-thirds is written as $\frac{2}{3}$, or $^2/_3$, or even 2/3.
  This can be read as *two divided by three*, or as *two parts out of three*.

- Fractions are concise ways of stating proportions: *three out of four* is the same as $\frac{3}{4}$. The same proportional value can be expressed by many equivalent fractions.

  For example, $\frac{3}{4} = \frac{6}{8} = \frac{12}{16} = \frac{75}{100}$. To create these equivalent fractions you can multiply (or divide) the numerator and the denominator by the same value. As long as the numerator and the denominator are multiplied by the same amount the resulting fraction will be equivalent to what you started with.

Multiplying fractions

- To multiply a whole number by a fraction the numerator only is multiplied by the whole number. If the fraction is less than one the result will be less than the whole number you started with.

  For example, $6 \times \frac{2}{3} = \frac{6 \times 2}{3} = \frac{12}{3} = 4$. Four is less than six because $\frac{2}{3}$ is less than one.

- To multiply two fractions you first multiply the two numerators and then multiply the two denominators.

  For example, $\frac{2}{3} \times \frac{3}{5} = \frac{2 \times 3}{3 \times 5} = \frac{6}{15}$, or $\frac{3}{4} \times \frac{1}{5} = \frac{3 \times 1}{4 \times 5} = \frac{3}{20}$. Sometimes both the numerator and the denominator can be divided by the same number to obtain an equivalent fraction that is said to be in a simpler form. This can be done with the first of the two examples above. $\frac{6}{15} = \frac{6 \div 3}{15 \div 3} = \frac{2}{5}$. Notice that *both* the numerator and the denominator are divided by the *same* number, ie 3.

Dividing fractions

- To divide one fraction by another, invert the second fraction and then multiply.

  For example, $\frac{4}{5} \div \frac{1}{2} = \frac{4}{5} \times \frac{2}{1} = \frac{8}{5}$; or $6 \div \frac{2}{3} = 6 \times \frac{2}{3} = \frac{18}{2} = 9$

- To find the *reciprocal* of a fraction simply tip it upside down.

  For example, the reciprocal of $\frac{4}{5}$ is $\frac{5}{4}$. Note that dividing by a fraction is the same as multiplying by its reciprocal.

Adding and subtracting fractions

- To add or subtract fractions they must have the same denominator. If the fractions do not have the same denominator then you must find equivalent fractions with a common denominator before you can add or subtract them.

  For example, $\frac{3}{5} + \frac{1}{5} = \frac{4}{5}$. This is straightforward because both fractions are fifths. Notice that only the numerators are added (or subtracted).

- If we wish to add $\frac{1}{2}$ and $\frac{3}{5}$ then we need to find equivalent fractions with a *common denominator*. In this case both fractions can be changed to *tenths*.

  So we have $\frac{1}{2} = \frac{5}{10}$, and $\frac{3}{5} = \frac{6}{10}$. Therefore $\frac{1}{2} + \frac{3}{5} = \frac{5}{10} + \frac{6}{10} = \frac{11}{10} = 1\frac{1}{10}$

Converting fractions to decimals and percentages

- To change a fraction to a decimal divide the numerator by the denominator. This is best done using a calculator.

  For example, $\frac{2}{5} = 2 \div 5 = 0.40$

- To change a fraction into a percentage first of all change it into a decimal and then move the decimal point two places to the right (ie multiply by 100).

  For example, $\frac{3}{8} = 3 \div 8 = 0.375 = 37.5\%$

Dealing with decimals

- Decimals are similar to fractions in that they are used to represent parts of a whole. The position of a digit to the left or right of the decimal point determines the value of the digit. The further left the larger the value, while the further to the right the less the value of the digit. Each move to the left or the right increases or decreases the place value by a factor of ten.

  For example, in the number 24.375 the digits have the following values:

  The 2 is equivalent to two tens $\qquad$ $2 \times 10 = 20$

  The 4 is equivalent to four units or four ones $\qquad$ $4 \times 1 = 4$

  The 3 is equivalent to three tenths $\qquad$ $3 \times \frac{1}{10} = \frac{3}{10}$, or 0.3

  The 7 is equivalent to seven hundredths $\qquad$ $7 \times \frac{1}{100} = \frac{7}{100}$, or 0.07

  The 5 is equivalent to five thousandths $\qquad$ $5 \times \frac{1}{1000} = \frac{5}{1000}$, or 0.005

- To change a decimal to a fraction use the number without the decimal point as the numerator. The denominator is the place value of the digit furthest to the right.

  For example, $0.025 = \frac{25}{1000}$ because the five occupies the thousandths place value.

  Similarly, $0.33 = \frac{33}{100}$, $0.5 = \frac{5}{10}$, $2.75 = \frac{275}{100} = 2\frac{75}{100} = 2\frac{3}{4}$.

Adding and subtracting decimals

- To add and subtract decimals the only rule is to keep the decimals points aligned. It can be helpful to think you are dealing with money when operating with decimals. Calculations with decimals are often best handled using a calculator.

  For example,

  $$\begin{array}{r} 0.12 \\ +2.507 \\ \hline 2.627 \end{array} \qquad \begin{array}{r} 2.75 \\ -0.975 \\ \hline 1.775 \end{array}$$

Multiplying and dividing decimals

- To multiply two decimals proceed by ignoring the decimal points. In the final answer the decimal point is positioned such that the number of digits to the right is the same as the total number of digits to the right in the two numbers being multiplied.

	1	.	2	5		two decimal places
×	0	.	3	7	5	three decimal places
			6	2	5	
		8	7	5	0	
	3	7	5	0	0	
0.	4	6	8	7	5	five decimal places

- To divide by decimals express them as a fraction, and then remove the decimal point in the numerator and denominator by multiplying both by 10, 100, 1000, or whatever is necessary to remove the decimal places. Remember to make sure you multiply both numerator and denominator by the same amount.

  For example $4 \div 0.25$ is the same as $\frac{4}{0.25}$. Multiplying both numerator and

Practical statistics for the health sciences

denominator by 100 will remove the decimal in the denominator. So we get
$$\frac{4 \times 100}{0.25 \times 100} = \frac{400}{25} = 16$$

- To change a decimal to a percentage involves multiplying by 100; ie moving the decimal point two places to the right.
  For example 0.25 = 25%; 0.575 = 57.5%; and 1.50 = 150%
- To convert a percentage to a decimal the percentage sign is removed and the resulting number divided by 100; ie the decimal point is moved two places to the left.
  For example, 75% = 75 = 0.75; 12.5% = 12.5 = 0.125; 1.5% = 1.5 = 0.015
- Arithmetic operations with decimals are best handled using a calculator. What needs to be remembered is that when you multiply by a number less than one you will end up with less than what you started with. On the other hand when you divide by a number less than one you will end up with more than what you started with.

Review of algebraic operations

Finding solutions to equations

- Whatever you do to one side of an equation you must do to the other in order to preserve the equality.
- When you want to get rid of something that has been added (or subtracted) to (or from) one side of an equation, move it to the other side and reverse the sign.
  For example, $5 + X = 16$ is equivalent to $X = 16 - 5$. The five has been subtracted from both sides of the equation leaving X on one side by itself.
  Another example: $X - 8 = 12$ is equivalent to $X = 12 + 8$.
- If you want to get rid of something that is in the numerator of one side of an equation move it to the other side and place it in the denominator.
  For example, $2X = 9$ is equivalent to $X = \frac{9}{2}$.
- If you want to get rid of something that is in the denominator move it to the other side of the equation and place it in the numerator.
  For example, $\frac{X}{3} = 9$ is equivalent to $X = 9 \times 3$.
- With more complex equations proceed one step at a time remembering to multiply (or divide) everything on the other side of the equation. The examples below show this.
  $4.5X - 3 = 6$ is equivalent to $4.5X = 6 + 3$, which in turn gives $X = \frac{6+3}{4.5}$ $= \frac{9}{4.5} = 2$.
  $\frac{X+4}{3} = 5$ gives $X + 4 = 5 \times 3 = 15$ which in turn gives $X = 15 - 4 = 11$.

Review of exponents and square roots

Notation

- Whenever a number is multiplied by itself the notation consists of placing an *exponent* to the right, and slightly above, the number concerned.
  For example, $3 \times 3 \times 3 \times 3$ is written as 3^4 and is read as 3 to the power 4.
  For negative numbers the same applies: $-5(-5)(-5)$ is written -5^3 or $(-5)^3$.

Properties of exponents

- Any number raised to the power of zero equals 1.
  For example, $2^0 = 1$; $-3^0 = 1$; $52.5^0 = 1$.
- Any number raised to the power one is equal to itself.
  For example, $6^1 = 6$; $-4.5^1 = -4.5$; $a^1 = a$.
- The exponent applies only to the number immediately preceding it.
  For example, ab^3 means $a \times b \times b \times b$, and x^2y means $x \times x \times y$.
- If an exponent applies to a bracket then the computations within the brackets should be carried out, where possible, before the exponential computation.
  For example, $(4 + 3)^3 = (7)^3 = 343$; $(4 - 7)^3 = -3^3 = -27$.
  Notice that $(4 + 3)^3$ is not the same as $4^3 + 3^3$; this is a common mistake.
  $4^3 + 3^3 = 64 + 27 = 91$. This means that $a^3 + b^3 \neq (a + b)^3$.
- When a fraction is raised to a certain power then both numerator and denominator are raised to the same power.
  For example, $\left(\frac{2}{3}\right)^2 = \frac{2^2}{3^2} = \frac{4}{9}$.

Square roots

- The square root is only taken for numbers under the square root sign (radical).
  For example, $\sqrt{16} = 4$, but $\sqrt{9} + 7 = 3 + 7 = 10$.
- Taking the square root of a number is the opposite (inverse) of raising a number to the second power, ie squaring
  For example, $\sqrt{4^2} = 4$, or more generally, $\sqrt{a^2} = a$.
- Computations involving addition and subtraction under the square root sign must be carried out before taking the square root.
  For example, $\sqrt{3 + 6} = \sqrt{9} = 3$. Note that this is not the same as $\sqrt{3} + \sqrt{6}$. This latter expression equals $1.732 + 2.449 = 4.181$.
- Computations involving multiplication and division may be carried out either before or after taking the square root.
  For example, $\sqrt{4 \times 9} = \sqrt{36} = 6$ may also be done as $\sqrt{4} \times \sqrt{9} = 2 \times 3 = 6$.
  This means that $\sqrt{a} \times \sqrt{b} = \sqrt{ab}$.
  Also, $\sqrt{16 \div 4}$ can be written as $\sqrt{\frac{16}{4}} = \sqrt{4} = 2$. Or, $\sqrt{\frac{16}{4}} = \frac{\sqrt{16}}{\sqrt{4}} = \frac{4}{2} = 2$.
- In algebraic expressions, to undo the taking of a square root you should square.
  For example, $\sqrt{X + 3} = 4$ may be solved for X by squaring both sides:
  $(\sqrt{X + 3})^2 = 4^2$ gives $X + 3 = 16$. Therefore $X = 13$.

Practical statistics for the health sciences

Solutions to self-assessment test

Part 1

1 4 **2** 12 **3** 6 **4** 12 **5** –18 **6** 12 **7** –18 **8** –36 **9** –3 **10** 7 **11** –4 **12** 8

Part 2

1 $\frac{4}{100}$, $\frac{4}{10}$, or $\frac{2}{5}$ **2** 60% **3** 0.625 **4** $\frac{6}{7}$ **5** 3.9 **6** $\frac{6}{20}$, or $\frac{3}{10}$ **7** $\frac{6}{24}$, or $\frac{1}{4}$ **8** 1.38

9 $\frac{8}{15}$ **10** 7 **11** 18 **12** 24

Part 3

1 13 **2** 16 **3** 23 **4** 6 **5** 8 **6** 24 **7** 36 **8** 7 **9** 3 **10** 26 **11** 20 **12** 8

Part 4

1 25 **2** 6 **3** 43 **4** 49 **5** 3 **6** 8 **7** –32 **8** 81 **9** 15 **10** 9 **11** 20; **12** –72

Appendix 3
Statistical tables

Table 1 Binomial probabilities — $\binom{n}{x} p^x(1-p)^{n-x}$

For a given combination of n and p the tabled entry indicates the probability of obtaining a specified value of x. For $p \leq 0.50$ read p across the top heading and both n and x down the *left* margin. For $p \geq 0.50$ read p across the bottom heading and both n and x up the *right* margin.

n	x	0.05	0.10	0.15	0.20	0.25	0.30	0.35	0.40	0.45	0.50		
2	0	0.9025	0.8100	0.7225	0.6400	0.5625	0.4900	0.4225	0.3600	0.3025	0.2500	2	
	1	0.0950	0.1800	0.2550	0.3200	0.3750	0.4200	0.4550	0.4800	0.4950	0.5000	1	
	2	0.0025	0.0100	0.0225	0.0400	0.0625	0.0900	0.1225	0.1600	0.2025	0.2500	0	2
3	0	0.8574	0.7290	0.6141	0.5120	0.4219	0.3430	0.2746	0.2160	0.1664	0.1250	3	
	1	0.1354	0.2430	0.3251	0.3840	0.4219	0.4410	0.4436	0.4320	0.4084	0.3750	2	
	2	0.0071	0.0270	0.0574	0.0960	0.1406	0.1890	0.2389	0.2880	0.3341	0.3750	1	
	3	0.0001	0.0010	0.0034	0.0080	0.0156	0.0270	0.0429	0.0640	0.0911	0.1250	0	3
4	0	0.8145	0.6561	0.5220	0.4096	0.3164	0.2401	0.1785	0.1296	0.0915	0.0625	4	
	1	0.1715	0.2916	0.3685	0.4096	0.4219	0.4116	0.3845	0.3456	0.2995	0.2500	3	
	2	0.0135	0.0486	0.0975	0.1536	0.2109	0.2646	0.3105	0.3456	0.3675	0.3750	2	
	3	0.0005	0.0036	0.0115	0.0256	0.0469	0.0756	0.1115	0.1536	0.2005	0.2500	1	
	4	0.0000	0.0001	0.0005	0.0016	0.0039	0.0081	0.0150	0.0256	0.0410	0.0625	0	4
5	0	0.7738	0.5905	0.4437	0.3277	0.2373	0.1681	0.1160	0.0778	0.0503	0.0312	5	
	1	0.2036	0.3280	0.3915	0.4096	0.3955	0.3601	0.3124	0.2592	0.2059	0.1562	4	
	2	0.0214	0.0729	0.1382	0.2048	0.2637	0.3087	0.3364	0.3456	0.3369	0.3125	3	
	3	0.0011	0.0081	0.0244	0.0512	0.0879	0.1323	0.1811	0.2304	0.2757	0.3125	2	
	4	0.0000	0.0004	0.0022	0.0064	0.0146	0.0283	0.0488	0.0768	0.1128	0.1562	1	
	5		0.0000	0.0001	0.0003	0.0010	0.0024	0.0053	0.0102	0.0185	0.0312	0	5
6	0	0.7351	0.5314	0.3771	0.2621	0.1780	0.1176	0.0754	0.0467	0.0277	0.0156	6	
	1	0.2321	0.3543	0.3993	0.3932	0.3560	0.3025	0.2437	0.1866	0.1359	0.0937	5	
	2	0.0305	0.0984	0.1762	0.2458	0.2966	0.3241	0.3280	0.3110	0.2780	0.2344	4	
	3	0.0021	0.0146	0.0415	0.0819	0.1318	0.1852	0.2355	0.2765	0.3032	0.3125	3	
	4	0.0001	0.0012	0.0055	0.0154	0.0330	0.0595	0.0951	0.1382	0.1861	0.2344	2	
	5	0.0000	0.0001	0.0004	0.0015	0.0044	0.0102	0.0205	0.0369	0.0609	0.0937	1	
	6		0.0000	0.0000	0.0001	0.0002	0.0007	0.0018	0.0041	0.0083	0.0156	0	6
7	0	0.6983	0.4783	0.3206	0.2097	0.1335	0.0824	0.0490	0.0280	0.0152	0.0078	7	
	1	0.2573	0.3720	0.3960	0.3670	0.3115	0.2471	0.1848	0.1306	0.0872	0.0547	6	
	2	0.0406	0.1240	0.2097	0.2753	0.3115	0.3177	0.2985	0.2613	0.2140	0.1641	5	
	3	0.0036	0.0230	0.0617	0.1147	0.1730	0.2269	0.2679	0.2903	0.2918	0.2734	4	
	4	0.0002	0.0026	0.0109	0.0287	0.0577	0.0972	0.1442	0.1935	0.2388	0.2734	3	
	5	0.0000	0.0002	0.0012	0.0043	0.0115	0.0250	0.0466	0.0774	0.1172	0.1641	2	
	6		0.0000	0.0001	0.0004	0.0013	0.0036	0.0084	0.0172	0.0320	0.0547	1	
	7			0.0000	0.0000	0.0001	0.0002	0.0006	0.0016	0.0037	0.0078	0	7
8	0	0.6634	0.4305	0.2725	0.1678	0.1001	0.0576	0.0319	0.0168	0.0084	0.0039	8	
	1	0.2739	0.3826	0.3847	0.3355	0.2670	0.1977	0.1373	0.0896	0.0548	0.0312	7	
	2	0.0515	0.1488	0.2376	0.2936	0.3115	0.2965	0.2587	0.2090	0.1569	0.1094	6	
	3	0.0054	0.0331	0.0839	0.1468	0.2076	0.2541	0.2786	0.2787	0.2568	0.2187	5	
	4	0.0004	0.0046	0.0185	0.0459	0.0865	0.1361	0.1875	0.2322	0.2627	0.2734	4	
	5	0.0000	0.0004	0.0026	0.0092	0.0231	0.0467	0.0808	0.1239	0.1719	0.2187	3	
	6		0.0000	0.0002	0.0011	0.0038	0.0100	0.0217	0.0413	0.0703	0.1094	2	
	7			0.0000	0.0001	0.0004	0.0012	0.0033	0.0079	0.0164	0.0312	1	
	8				0.0000	0.0000	0.0001	0.0002	0.0007	0.0017	0.0039	0	8
		0.95	0.90	0.85	0.80	0.75	0.70	0.65	0.60	0.55	0.50	x	n

Table 1 Binomial probabilities (continued)

x	n	0.05	0.10	0.15	0.20	0.25	0.30	0.35	0.40	0.45	0.50		
9	0	0.6302	0.3874	0.2316	0.1342	0.0751	0.0404	0.0207	0.0101	0.0046	0.0020	9	
	1	0.2985	0.3874	0.3679	0.3020	0.2253	0.1556	0.1004	0.0605	0.0339	0.0176	8	
	2	0.0629	0.1722	0.2597	0.3020	0.3003	0.2668	0.2162	0.1612	0.1110	0.0703	7	
	3	0.0077	0.0446	0.1069	0.1762	0.2336	0.2668	0.2716	0.2508	0.2119	0.1641	6	
	4	0.0006	0.0074	0.0283	0.0661	0.1168	0.1715	0.2194	0.2508	0.2600	0.2461	5	
	5	0.0000	0.0008	0.0050	0.0165	0.0389	0.0735	0.1181	0.1672	0.2128	0.2461	4	
	6		0.0001	0.0006	0.0028	0.0087	0.0210	0.0424	0.0743	0.1160	0.1641	3	
	7		0.0000	0.0000	0.0003	0.0012	0.0039	0.0098	0.0212	0.0407	0.0703	2	
	8				0.0000	0.0001	0.0004	0.0013	0.0035	0.0083	0.0176	1	
	9					0.0000	0.0000	0.0001	0.0003	0.0008	0.0020	0	9
10	0	0.5987	0.3487	0.1969	0.1074	0.0563	0.0282	0.0135	0.0060	0.0025	0.0010	10	
	1	0.3151	0.3874	0.3474	0.2684	0.1877	0.1211	0.0725	0.0403	0.0207	0.0098	9	
	2	0.0746	0.1937	0.2759	0.3020	0.2816	0.2335	0.1757	0.1209	0.0763	0.0439	8	
	3	0.0105	0.0574	0.1298	0.2013	0.2503	0.2668	0.2522	0.2150	0.1665	0.1172	7	
	4	0.0010	0.0112	0.0401	0.0881	0.1460	0.2001	0.2377	0.2508	0.2384	0.2051	6	
	5	0.0001	0.0015	0.0085	0.0264	0.0584	0.1029	0.1536	0.2007	0.2340	0.2461	5	
	6	0.0000	0.0001	0.0012	0.0055	0.0162	0.0368	0.0689	0.1115	0.1596	0.2051	4	
	7		0.0000	0.0001	0.0008	0.0031	0.0090	0.0212	0.0425	0.0746	0.1172	3	
	8			0.0000	0.0001	0.0004	0.0014	0.0043	0.0106	0.0229	0.0439	2	
	9				0.0000	0.0000	0.0001	0.0005	0.0016	0.0042	0.0098	1	
	10						0.0000	0.0000	0.0001	0.0003	0.0010	0	10
11	0	0.5688	0.3138	0.1673	0.0859	0.0422	0.0198	0.0088	0.0036	0.0014	0.0005	11	
	1	0.3293	0.3835	0.3248	0.2362	0.1549	0.0932	0.0518	0.0266	0.0125	0.0054	10	
	2	0.0867	0.2131	0.2866	0.2953	0.2581	0.1998	0.1395	0.0887	0.0513	0.0269	9	
	3	0.0137	0.0710	0.1517	0.2215	0.2581	0.2568	0.2254	0.1774	0.1259	0.0806	8	
	4	0.0014	0.0158	0.0536	0.1107	0.1721	0.2201	0.2428	0.2365	0.2060	0.1611	7	
	5	0.0001	0.0025	0.0132	0.0388	0.0803	0.1321	0.1830	0.2207	0.2360	0.2256	6	
	6	0.0000	0.0003	0.0023	0.0097	0.0268	0.0566	0.0985	0.1471	0.1931	0.2256	5	
	7		0.0000	0.0003	0.0017	0.0064	0.0173	0.0379	0.0701	0.1128	0.1611	4	
	8			0.0000	0.0002	0.0011	0.0037	0.0102	0.0234	0.0462	0.0806	3	
	9				0.0000	0.0001	0.0005	0.0018	0.0052	0.0126	0.0269	2	
	10						0.0000	0.0002	0.0007	0.0021	0.0054	1	
	11							0.0000	0.0000	0.0002	0.0005	0	11
12	0	0.5404	0.2824	0.1422	0.0687	0.0317	0.0138	0.0057	0.0022	0.0008	0.0002	12	
	1	0.3413	0.3766	0.3012	0.2062	0.1267	0.0712	0.0368	0.0174	0.0075	0.0029	11	
	2	0.0988	0.2301	0.2924	0.2835	0.2323	0.1678	0.1088	0.0639	0.0339	0.0161	10	
	3	0.0173	0.0852	0.1720	0.2362	0.2581	0.2397	0.1954	0.1419	0.0923	0.0537	9	
	4	0.0021	0.0213	0.0683	0.1329	0.1936	0.2311	0.2367	0.2128	0.1700	0.1208	8	
	5	0.0002	0.0038	0.0193	0.0532	0.1032	0.1585	0.2039	0.2270	0.2225	0.1934	7	
	6	0.0000	0.0005	0.0040	0.0155	0.0401	0.0792	0.1281	0.1766	0.2124	0.2256	6	
	7		0.0000	0.0006	0.0033	0.0115	0.0291	0.0591	0.1009	0.1489	0.1934	5	
	8			0.0001	0.0005	0.0024	0.0078	0.0199	0.0420	0.0762	0.1208	4	
	9			0.0000	0.0001	0.0004	0.0015	0.0048	0.0125	0.0277	0.0537	3	
	10					0.0000	0.0002	0.0008	0.0025	0.0068	0.0161	2	
	11						0.0000	0.0001	0.0003	0.0010	0.0029	1	
	12							0.0000	0.0000	0.0001	0.0002	0	12
		0.95	0.90	0.85	0.80	0.75	0.70	0.65	0.60	0.55	0.50	x	n

Practical statistics for the health sciences

Table 1 Binomial probabilities (continued)

n	x	0.05	0.10	0.15	0.20	0.25	0.30	0.35	0.40	0.45	0.50	
13	0	0.5133	0.2542	0.1209	0.0550	0.0238	0.0097	0.0037	0.0013	0.0004	0.0001	13
	1	0.3512	0.3672	0.2774	0.1787	0.1029	0.0540	0.0259	0.0113	0.0045	0.0016	12
	2	0.1109	0.2448	0.2937	0.2680	0.2059	0.1388	0.0836	0.0453	0.0220	0.0095	11
	3	0.0214	0.0997	0.1900	0.2457	0.2517	0.2181	0.1651	0.1107	0.0660	0.0349	10
	4	0.0028	0.0277	0.0838	0.1535	0.2097	0.2337	0.2222	0.1845	0.1350	0.0873	9
	5	0.0003	0.0055	0.0266	0.0691	0.1258	0.1803	0.2154	0.2214	0.1989	0.1571	8
	6	0.0000	0.0008	0.0063	0.0230	0.0559	0.1030	0.1546	0.1968	0.2169	0.2095	7
	7		0.0001	0.0011	0.0058	0.0186	0.0442	0.0833	0.1312	0.1775	0.2095	6
	8		0.0000	0.0001	0.0011	0.0047	0.0142	0.0336	0.0656	0.1089	0.1571	5
	9			0.0000	0.0001	0.0009	0.0034	0.0101	0.0243	0.0495	0.0873	4
	10				0.0000	0.0001	0.0006	0.0022	0.0065	0.0162	0.0349	3
	11					0.0000	0.0001	0.0003	0.0012	0.0036	0.0095	2
	12						0.0000	0.0000	0.0001	0.0005	0.0016	1
	13								0.0000	0.0000	0.0001	0 13
14	0	0.4877	0.2288	0.1028	0.0440	0.0178	0.0068	0.0024	0.0008	0.0002	0.0001	14
	1	0.3593	0.3559	0.2539	0.1539	0.0832	0.0407	0.0181	0.0073	0.0027	0.0009	13
	2	0.1229	0.2570	0.2912	0.2501	0.1802	0.1134	0.0634	0.0317	0.0141	0.0056	12
	3	0.0259	0.1142	0.2056	0.2501	0.2402	0.1943	0.1366	0.0845	0.0462	0.0222	11
	4	0.0037	0.0349	0.0998	0.1720	0.2202	0.2290	0.2022	0.1549	0.1040	0.0611	10
	5	0.0004	0.0078	0.0352	0.0860	0.1468	0.1963	0.2178	0.2066	0.1701	0.1222	9
	6	0.0000	0.0013	0.0093	0.0322	0.0734	0.1262	0.1759	0.2066	0.2088	0.1833	8
	7		0.0002	0.0019	0.0092	0.0280	0.0618	0.1082	0.1574	0.1952	0.2095	7
	8		0.0000	0.0003	0.0020	0.0082	0.0232	0.0510	0.0918	0.1398	0.1833	6
	9			0.0000	0.0003	0.0018	0.0066	0.0183	0.0408	0.0762	0.1222	5
	10				0.0000	0.0003	0.0014	0.0049	0.0136	0.0312	0.0611	4
	11					0.0000	0.0002	0.0010	0.0033	0.0093	0.0222	3
	12						0.0000	0.0001	0.0005	0.0019	0.0056	2
	13							0.0000	0.0001	0.0002	0.0009	1
	14								0.0000	0.0000	0.0001	0 14
15	0	0.4633	0.2059	0.0874	0.0352	0.0134	0.0047	0.0016	0.0005	0.0001	0.0000	15
	1	0.3658	0.3432	0.2312	0.1319	0.0668	0.0305	0.0126	0.0047	0.0016	0.0005	14
	2	0.1348	0.2669	0.2856	0.2309	0.1559	0.0916	0.0476	0.0219	0.0090	0.0032	13
	3	0.0307	0.1285	0.2184	0.2501	0.2252	0.1700	0.1110	0.0634	0.0318	0.0139	12
	4	0.0049	0.0428	0.1156	0.1876	0.2252	0.2186	0.1792	0.1268	0.0780	0.0417	11
	5	0.0006	0.0105	0.0449	0.1032	0.1651	0.2061	0.2123	0.1859	0.1404	0.0916	10
	6	0.0000	0.0019	0.0132	0.0430	0.0917	0.1472	0.1906	0.2066	0.1914	0.1527	9
	7		0.0003	0.0030	0.0138	0.0393	0.0811	0.1319	0.1771	0.2013	0.1964	8
	8		0.0000	0.0005	0.0035	0.0131	0.0348	0.0710	0.1181	0.1647	0.1964	7
	9			0.0001	0.0007	0.0034	0.0116	0.0298	0.0612	0.1048	0.1527	6
	10			0.0000	0.0001	0.0007	0.0030	0.0096	0.0245	0.0515	0.0916	5
	11				0.0000	0.0001	0.0006	0.0024	0.0074	0.0191	0.0417	4
	12					0.0000	0.0001	0.0004	0.0016	0.0052	0.0139	3
	13						0.0000	0.0001	0.0003	0.0010	0.0032	2
	14							0.0000	0.0000	0.0001	0.0005	1
	15									0.0000	0.0000	0 15
		0.95	0.90	0.85	0.80	0.75	0.70	0.65	0.60	0.55	0.50	x n

Table 1 Binomial probabilities (continued)

n	x	0.05	0.10	0.15	0.20	0.25	0.30	0.35	0.40	0.45	0.50	
20	0	0.3585	0.1216	0.0388	0.0115	0.0032	0.0008	0.0002	0.0000	0.0000	0.0000	20
	1	0.3774	0.2702	0.1368	0.0576	0.0211	0.0068	0.0020	0.0005	0.0001	0.0000	19
	2	0.1887	0.2852	0.2293	0.1369	0.0669	0.0278	0.0100	0.0031	0.0008	0.0002	18
	3	0.0596	0.1901	0.2428	0.2054	0.1339	0.0716	0.0323	0.0123	0.0040	0.0011	17
	4	0.0133	0.0898	0.1821	0.2182	0.1897	0.1304	0.0738	0.0350	0.0139	0.0046	16
	5	0.0022	0.0319	0.1028	0.1746	0.2023	0.1789	0.1272	0.0746	0.0365	0.0148	15
	6	0.0003	0.0089	0.0454	0.1091	0.1686	0.1916	0.1712	0.1244	0.0746	0.0370	14
	7	0.0000	0.0020	0.0160	0.0545	0.1124	0.1643	0.1844	0.1659	0.1221	0.0739	13
	8		0.0004	0.0046	0.0222	0.0609	0.1144	0.1614	0.1797	0.1623	0.1201	12
	9		0.0001	0.0011	0.0074	0.0271	0.0654	0.1158	01597	0.1771	0.1602	11
	10		0.0000	0.0002	0.0020	0.0099	0.0308	0.0686	0.1171	0.1593	0.1762	10
	11			0.0000	0.0005	0.0030	0.0120	0.0336	0.0710	0.1185	0.1602	9
	12				0.0001	0.0008	0.0039	0.0136	0.0355	0.0727	0.1201	8
	13				0.0000	0.0002	0.0010	0.0045	0.0146	0.0366	0.0739	7
	14					0.0000	0.0002	0.0012	0.0049	0.0150	0.0370	6
	15						0.0000	0.0003	0.0013	0.0049	0.0148	5
	16							0.0000	0.0003	0.0013	0.0046	4
	17								0.0000	0.0002	0.0011	3
	18									0.0000	0.0002	2
	19										0.0000	1
	20											0 20
		0.95	0.90	0.85	0.80	0.75	0.70	0.65	0.60	0.55	0.50	x n

Table 2 Areas under the standard normal probability distribution

Each entry in the body of the table represents the area under the standardised normal distribution between the mean ($z = 0$) and the specified z-score.
Negative z-values refer to points on the left half of the distribution.

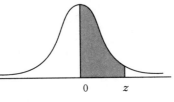

z	.00	.01	.02	.03	.04	.05	.06	.07	.08	.09
0.0	.0000	.0040	.0080	.0120	.0160	.0199	.0239	.0279	.0319	.0359
0.1	.0398	.0438	.0478	.0517	.0557	.0596	.0636	.0675	.0714	.0753
0.2	.0793	.0832	.0871	.0910	.0948	.0987	.1026	.1064	.1103	.1141
0.3	.1179	.1217	.1255	.1293	.1331	.1368	.1406	.1443	.1480	.1517
0.4	.1554	.1591	.1628	.1664	.1700	.1736	.1772	.1808	.1844	.1879
0.5	.1915	.1950	.1985	.2019	.2054	.2088	.2123	.2157	.2190	.2224
0.6	.2257	.2291	.2324	.2357	.2389	.2422	.2454	.2486	.2518	.2549
0.7	.2580	.2612	.2642	.2673	.2704	.2734	.2764	.2794	.2823	.2852
0.8	.2881	.2910	.2939	.2967	.2995	.3023	.3051	.3078	.3106	.3133
0.9	.3159	.3186	.3212	.3238	.3264	.3289	.3315	.3340	.3365	.3389
1.0	.3413	.3438	.3461	.3485	.3508	.3531	.3554	.3577	.3599	.3621
1.1	.3643	.3665	.3686	.3708	.3729	.3749	.3770	.3790	.3810	.3830
1.2	.3849	.3869	.3888	.3907	.3925	.3944	.3962	.3980	.3997	.4015
1.3	.4032	.4049	.4066	.4082	.4099	.4115	.4131	.4147	.4162	.4177
1.4	.4192	.4207	.4222	.4236	.4251	.4265	.4279	.4292	.4306	.4319
1.5	.4332	.4345	.4357	.4370	.4382	.4394	.4406	.4418	.4429	.4441
1.6	.4452	.4463	.4474	.4484	.4495	.4505	.4515	.4525	.4535	.4545
1.7	.4554	.4564	.4573	.4582	.4591	.4599	.4608	.4616	.4625	.4633
1.8	.4641	.4649	.4656	.4664	.4671	.4678	.4686	.4693	.4699	.4706
1.9	.4713	.4719	.4726	.4732	.4738	.4744	.4750	.4756	.4761	.4767
2.0	.4772	.4778	.4783	.4788	.4793	.4798	.4803	.4808	.4812	.4817
2.1	.4821	.4826	.4830	.4834	.4838	.4842	.4846	.4850	.4854	.4857
2.2	.4861	.4864	.4868	.4871	.4875	.4878	.4881	.4884	.4887	.4890
2.3	.4893	.4896	.4898	.4901	.4904	.4906	.4909	.4911	.4913	.4916
2.4	.4918	.4920	.4922	.4925	.4927	.4929	.4931	.4932	.4934	.4936
2.5	.4938	.4940	.4941	.4943	.4945	.4946	.4948	.4949	.4951	.4952
2.6	.4953	.4955	.4956	.4957	.4959	.4960	.4961	.4962	.4963	.4964
2.7	.4965	.4966	.4967	.4968	.4969	.4970	.4971	.4972	.4973	.4974
2.8	.4974	.4975	.4976	.4977	.4977	.4978	.4979	.4979	.4980	.4981
2.9	.4981	.4982	.4982	.4983	.4984	.4984	.4985	.4985	.4986	.4986
3.0	.49865	.49869	.49874	.49878	.49882	.49886	.49889	.49893	.49897	.49900
3.1	.49903	.49906	.49910	.49913	.49916	.49918	.49921	.49924	.49926	.49929
3.2	.49931	.49934	.49936	.49938	.49940	.49942	.49944	.49946	.49948	.49950
3.3	.49952	.49953	.49955	.49957	.49958	.49960	.49961	.49962	.49964	.49965
3.4	.49966	.49968	.49969	.49970	.49971	.49972	.49973	.49974	.49975	.49976
3.5	.49977	.49978	.49978	.49979	.49980	.49981	.49981	.49982	.49983	.49983
3.6	.49984	.49985	.49985	.49986	.49986	.49987	.49987	.49988	.49988	.49989
3.7	.49989	.49990	.49990	.49990	.49991	.49991	.49992	.49992	.49992	.49992
3.8	.49993	.49993	.49993	.49994	.49994	.49994	.49994	.49995	.49995	.49995
3.9	.49995	.49995	.49996	.49996	.49996	.49996	.49996	.49996	.49997	.49997

Table 3 Student's *t*-distribution

For a particular number of degrees of freedom each entry represents the critical value of *t* corresponding to a specified upper tail area α.

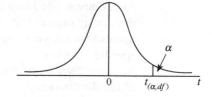

Degrees of freedom	Upper tail area					
	.25	.10	.05	.025	.01	.005
1	1.0000	3.0777	6.3138	12.7062	31.8207	63.6574
2	0.8165	1.8856	2.9200	4.3027	6.9646	9.9248
3	0.7649	1.6377	2.3534	3.1824	4.5407	5.8409
4	0.7407	1.5332	2.1318	2.7764	3.7469	4.6041
5	0.7267	1.4759	2.0150	2.5706	3.3649	4.0322
6	0.7176	1.4398	1.9432	2.4469	3.1427	3.7074
7	0.7111	1.4149	1.8946	2.3646	2.9980	3.4995
8	0.7064	1.3968	1.8595	2.3060	2.8965	3.3554
9	0.7027	1.3830	1.8331	2.2622	2.8214	3.2498
10	0.6998	1.3722	1.8125	2.2281	2.7638	3.1693
11	0.6974	1.3634	1.7959	2.2010	2.7181	3.1058
12	0.6955	1.3562	1.7823	2.1788	2.6810	3.0545
13	0.6938	1.3502	1.7709	2.1604	2.6503	3.0123
14	0.6924	1.3450	1.7613	2.1448	2.6245	2.9768
15	0.6912	1.3406	1.7531	2.1315	2.6025	2.9467
16	0.6901	1.3368	1.7459	2.1199	2.5835	2.9208
17	0.6892	1.3334	1.7396	2.1098	2.5669	2.8982
18	0.6884	1.3304	1.7341	2.1009	2.5524	2.8784
19	0.6876	1.3277	1.7291	2.0930	2.5395	2.8609
20	0.6870	1.3253	1.7247	2.0860	2.5280	2.8453
21	0.6864	1.3232	1.7207	2.0796	2.5177	2.8314
22	0.6858	1.3212	1.7171	2.0739	2.5083	2.8188
23	0.6853	1.3195	1.7139	2.0687	2.4999	2.8073
24	0.6848	1.3178	1.7109	2.0639	2.4922	2.7969
25	0.6844	1.3163	1.7081	2.0595	2.4851	2.7874
26	0.6840	1.3150	1.7056	2.0555	2.4786	2.7787
27	0.6837	1.3137	1.7033	2.0518	2.4727	2.7707
28	0.6834	1.3125	1.7011	2.0484	2.4671	2.7633
29	0.6830	1.3114	1.6991	2.0452	2.4620	2.7564
30	0.6828	1.3104	1.6973	2.0423	2.4573	2.7500
40	0.6807	1.3031	1.6839	2.0211	2.4233	2.7045
50	0.6794	1.2987	1.6759	2.0086	2.4033	2.6778
60	0.6786	1.2958	1.6706	2.0003	2.3901	2.6603
70	0.6780	1.2938	1.6669	1.9944	2.3808	2.6479
80	0.6776	1.2922	1.6641	1.9901	2.3739	2.6387
90	0.6772	1.2910	1.6620	1.9867	2.3685	2.6316
100	0.6770	1.2901	1.6602	1.9840	2.3642	2.6259
∞	0.6745	1.2816	1.6449	1.9600	2.3263	2.5758

Practical statistics for the health sciences

Table 4 Critical values of F for $\alpha = 0.01$

For a particular combination of numerator and denominator degrees of freedom, each entry in the body of the table represents the critical values of F corresponding to the specified upper tail area (α).

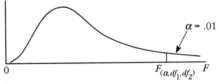

$\alpha = .01$

$F_{(\alpha, df_1, df_2)}$

Denom	Numerator df									
df	1	2	3	4	5	6	7	8	9	10
1	4052	4999	5403	5625	5764	5859	5928	5982	6022	6056
2	98.50	99.00	99.17	99.25	99.30	99.33	99.36	99.37	99.39	99.40
3	34.12	30.82	29.46	28.71	28.24	27.91	27.67	27.49	27.35	27.23
4	21.20	18.00	16.69	15.98	15.52	15.21	14.98	14.80	14.66	14.55
5	16.26	13.27	12.06	11.39	10.97	10.67	10.46	10.29	10.16	10.05
6	13.75	10.92	9.78	9.15	8.75	8.47	8.26	8.10	7.98	7.87
7	12.25	9.55	8.45	7.85	7.46	7.19	6.99	6.84	6.72	6.62
8	11.26	8.65	7.59	7.01	6.63	6.37	6.18	6.03	5.91	5.81
9	10.56	8.02	6.99	6.42	6.06	5.80	5.61	5.47	5.35	5.26
10	10.04	7.56	6.55	5.99	5.64	5.39	5.20	5.06	4.94	4.85
11	9.65	7.21	6.22	5.67	5.32	5.07	4.89	4.74	4.63	4.54
12	9.33	6.93	5.95	5.41	5.06	4.82	4.64	4.50	4.39	4.30
13	9.07	6.70	5.74	5.21	4.86	4.62	4.44	4.30	4.19	4.10
14	8.86	6.51	5.56	5.04	4.69	4.46	4.28	4.14	4.03	3.94
15	8.68	6.36	5.42	4.89	4.56	4.32	4.14	4.00	3.89	3.80
16	8.53	6.23	5.29	4.77	4.44	4.20	4.03	3.89	3.78	3.69
17	8.40	6.11	5.18	4.67	4.34	4.10	3.93	3.79	3.68	3.59
18	8.29	6.01	5.09	4.58	4.25	4.01	3.84	3.71	3.60	3.51
19	8.18	5.93	5.01	4.50	4.17	3.94	3.77	3.63	3.52	3.43
20	8.10	5.85	5.94	4.43	4.10	3.87	3.70	3.56	3.46	3.37
21	8.02	5.78	4.87	4.37	4.04	3.81	3.64	3.51	3.40	3.31
22	7.95	5.72	4.82	4.31	3.99	3.76	3.59	3.45	3.35	3.26
23	7.88	5.66	4.76	4.26	3.94	3.71	3.54	3.41	3.30	3.21
24	7.82	5.61	4.72	4.22	3.90	3.67	3.50	3.36	3.26	3.17
25	7.77	5.57	4.68	4.18	3.85	3.63	3.46	3.32	3.22	3.13
26	7.72	5.53	4.64	4.14	3.82	3.59	3.42	3.29	3.18	3.09
27	7.68	5.49	4.60	4.11	3.78	3.56	3.39	3.26	3.15	3.06
28	7.64	5.45	4.57	4.07	3.75	3.53	3.36	3.23	3.12	3.03
29	7.60	5.42	4.54	4.04	3.73	3.50	3.33	3.20	3.09	3.00
30	7.56	5.39	4.51	4.02	3.70	3.47	3.30	3.17	3.07	2.98
40	7.31	5.18	4.31	3.83	3.51	3.29	3.12	2.99	2.89	2.80
60	7.08	4.98	4.13	3.65	3.34	3.12	2.95	2.82	2.72	2.63
120	6.85	4.79	3.95	3.48	3.17	2.96	2.79	2.66	2.56	2.47
∞	6.63	4.61	3.78	3.32	3.02	2.80	2.64	2.51	2.41	2.32

Table 4 Critical values of F for $\alpha = 0.01$ (continued)

Denom df	Numerator df								
	12	15	20	24	30	40	60	120	∞
1	6106	6157	6209	6235	6261	6287	6313	6339	6366
2	99.42	99.43	99.45	99.46	99.47	99.47	99.48	99.49	99.50
3	27.05	26.87	26.69	26.60	26.50	26.41	26.32	26.22	26.13
4	14.37	14.20	14.02	13.93	13.84	13.75	13.65	13.56	13.46
5	9.89	9.72	9.55	9.47	9.38	9.29	9.20	9.11	9.02
6	7.72	7.56	7.40	7.31	7.23	7.14	7.06	6.97	6.88
7	6.47	6.31	6.16	6.07	5.99	5.91	5.82	5.74	5.65
8	5.67	5.52	5.36	5.28	5.20	5.12	5.03	4.95	4.86
9	5.11	4.96	4.81	4.73	4.65	4.57	4.48	4.40	4.31
10	4.71	4.56	4.41	4.33	4.25	4.17	4.08	4.00	3.91
11	4.40	4.25	4.10	4.02	3.94	3.86	3.78	3.69	3.60
12	4.16	4.01	3.86	3.78	3.70	3.62	3.54	3.45	3.36
13	3.96	3.82	3.66	3.59	3.51	3.43	3.34	3.25	3.17
14	3.80	3.66	3.51	3.43	3.35	3.27	3.18	3.09	3.00
15	3.67	3.52	3.37	3.29	3.21	3.13	3.05	2.96	2.87
16	3.55	3.41	3.26	3.18	3.10	3.02	2.93	2.84	2.75
17	3.46	3.31	3.16	3.08	3.00	2.92	2.83	2.75	2.65
18	3.37	3.23	3.08	3.00	2.92	2.84	2.75	2.66	2.57
19	3.30	3.15	3.00	2.92	2.84	2.76	2.67	2.58	2.49
20	3.23	3.09	2.94	2.86	2.78	2.69	2.61	2.52	2.42
21	3.17	3.03	2.88	2.80	2.72	2.64	2.55	2.46	2.36
22	3.12	2.98	2.83	2.75	2.67	2.58	2.50	2.40	2.31
23	3.07	2.93	2.78	2.70	2.62	2.54	2.45	2.35	2.26
24	3.03	2.89	2.74	2.66	2.58	2.49	2.40	2.31	2.21
25	2.99	2.85	2.70	2.62	2.54	2.45	2.36	2.27	2.17
26	2.96	2.81	2.66	2.58	2.50	2.42	2.33	2.23	2.13
27	2.93	2.78	2.63	2.55	2.47	2.38	2.29	2.20	2.10
28	2.90	2.75	2.60	2.52	2.44	2.35	2.26	2.17	2.06
29	2.87	2.73	2.57	2.49	2.41	2.33	2.23	2.14	2.03
30	2.84	2.70	2.55	2.47	2.39	2.30	2.21	2.11	2.01
40	2.66	2.52	2.37	2.29	2.20	2.11	2.02	1.92	1.80
60	2.50	2.35	2.20	2.12	2.03	1.94	1.84	1.73	1.60
120	2.34	2.19	2.03	1.95	1.86	1.76	1.66	1.53	1.38
∞	2.18	2.04	1.88	1.79	1.70	1.59	1.47	1.32	1.00

Practical statistics for the health sciences

Table 5 Critical values of F for $\alpha = 0.05$

For a particular combination of numerator and denominator degrees of freedom, each entry in the body of the table represents the critical values of F corresponding to the specified upper tail area (α).

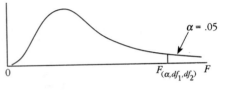

Denom	Numerator df									
df	1	2	3	4	5	6	7	8	9	10
1	161.40	199.50	215.70	224.60	230.20	234.00	236.80	238.90	240.50	241.90
2	18.51	19.00	19.16	19.25	19.30	19.33	19.35	19.37	19.38	19.40
3	10.13	9.55	9.28	9.12	9.01	8.94	8.89	8.85	8.81	8.79
4	7.71	6.94	6.59	6.39	6.26	6.16	6.09	6.04	6.00	5.96
5	6.61	5.79	5.41	5.19	5.05	4.95	4.88	4.82	4.77	4.74
6	5.99	5.14	4.76	4.53	4.39	4.28	4.21	4.15	4.10	4.06
7	5.59	4.74	4.35	4.12	3.97	3.87	3.79	3.73	3.68	3.64
8	5.32	4.46	4.07	3.84	3.69	3.58	3.50	3.44	3.39	3.35
9	5.12	4.26	3.86	3.63	3.48	3.37	3.29	3.23	3.18	3.14
10	4.96	4.10	3.71	3.48	3.33	3.22	3.14	3.07	3.02	2.98
11	4.84	3.98	3.59	3.36	3.20	3.09	3.01	2.95	2.90	2.85
12	4.75	3.89	3.49	3.26	3.11	3.00	2.91	2.85	2.80	2.75
13	4.67	3.81	3.41	3.18	3.03	2.92	2.83	2.77	2.71	2.67
14	4.60	3.74	3.34	3.11	2.96	2.85	2.76	2.70	2.65	2.60
15	4.54	3.68	3.29	3.06	2.90	2.79	2.71	2.64	2.59	2.54
16	4.49	3.63	3.24	3.01	2.85	2.74	2.66	2.59	2.54	2.49
17	4.45	3.59	3.20	2.96	2.81	2.70	2.61	2.55	2.49	2.45
18	4.41	3.55	3.16	2.93	2.77	2.66	2.58	2.51	2.46	2.41
19	4.38	3.52	3.13	2.90	2.74	2.63	2.54	2.48	2.42	2.38
20	4.35	3.49	3.10	2.87	2.71	2.60	2.51	2.45	2.39	2.35
21	4.32	3.47	3.07	2.84	2.68	2.57	2.49	2.42	2.37	2.32
22	4.30	3.44	3.05	2.82	2.66	2.55	2.46	2.40	2.34	2.30
23	4.28	3.42	3.03	2.80	2.64	2.53	2.44	2.37	2.32	2.27
24	4.26	3.40	3.01	2.78	2.62	2.51	2.42	2.36	2.30	2.25
25	4.24	3.39	2.99	2.76	2.60	2.49	2.40	2.34	2.28	2.24
26	4.23	3.37	2.98	2.74	2.59	2.47	2.39	2.32	2.27	2.22
27	4.21	3.35	2.96	2.73	2.57	2.46	2.37	2.31	2.25	2.20
28	4.20	3.34	2.95	2.71	2.56	2.45	2.36	2.29	2.24	2.19
29	4.18	3.33	2.93	2.70	2.55	2.43	2.35	2.28	2.22	2.18
30	4.17	3.32	2.92	2.69	2.53	2.42	2.33	2.27	2.21	2.16
40	4.08	3.23	2.84	2.61	2.45	2.34	2.25	2.18	2.12	2.08
60	4.00	3.15	2.76	2.53	2.37	2.25	2.17	2.10	2.04	1.99
120	3.92	3.07	2.68	2.45	2.29	2.17	2.09	2.02	1.96	1.91
∞	3.84	3.00	2.60	2.37	2.21	2.10	2.01	1.94	1.88	1.83

Table 5 Critical values of F for $\alpha = 0.05$ (continued)

Denom df	\multicolumn{9}{c}{Numerator df}
	12	15	20	24	30	40	60	120	∞
1	243.90	245.90	248.00	249.10	250.10	251.10	252.20	253.30	254.30
2	19.41	19.43	19.45	19.45	19.46	19.47	19.48	19.49	19.50
3	8.74	8.70	8.66	8.64	8.62	8.59	8.57	8.55	8.53
4	5.91	5.86	5.80	5.77	5.75	5.72	5.69	5.66	5.63
5	4.68	4.62	4.56	4.53	4.50	4.46	4.43	4.40	4.36
6	4.00	3.94	3.87	3.84	3.81	3.77	3.74	3.70	3.67
7	3.57	3.51	3.44	3.41	3.38	3.34	3.30	3.27	3.23
8	3.28	3.22	3.15	3.12	3.08	3.04	3.01	2.97	2.93
9	3.07	3.01	2.94	2.90	2.86	2.83	2.79	2.75	2.71
10	2.91	2.85	2.77	2.74	2.70	2.66	2.62	2.58	2.54
11	2.79	2.72	2.65	2.61	2.57	2.53	2.49	2.45	2.40
12	2.69	2.62	2.54	2.51	2.47	2.43	2.38	2.34	2.30
13	2.60	2.53	2.46	2.42	2.38	2.34	2.30	2.25	2.21
14	2.53	2.46	2.39	2.35	2.31	2.27	2.22	2.18	2.13
15	2.48	2.40	2.33	2.29	2.25	2.20	2.16	2.11	2.07
16	2.42	2.35	2.28	2.24	2.19	2.15	2.11	2.06	2.01
17	2.38	2.31	2.23	2.19	2.15	2.10	2.06	2.01	1.96
18	2.34	2.27	2.19	2.15	2.11	2.06	2.02	1.97	1.92
19	2.31	2.23	2.16	2.11	2.07	2.03	1.98	1.93	1.88
20	2.28	2.20	2.12	2.08	2.04	1.99	1.95	1.90	1.84
21	2.25	2.18	2.10	2.05	2.01	1.96	1.92	1.87	1.81
22	2.23	2.15	2.07	2.03	1.98	1.94	1.89	1.84	1.78
23	2.20	2.13	2.05	2.01	1.96	1.91	1.86	1.81	1.76
24	2.18	2.11	2.03	1.98	1.94	1.89	1.84	1.79	1.73
25	2.16	2.09	2.01	1.96	1.92	1.87	1.82	1.77	1.71
26	2.15	2.07	1.99	1.95	1.90	1.85	1.80	1.75	1.69
27	2.13	2.06	1.97	1.93	1.88	1.84	1.79	1.73	1.67
28	2.12	2.04	1.96	1.91	1.87	1.82	1.77	1.71	1.65
29	2.10	2.03	1.94	1.90	1.85	1.81	1.75	1.70	1.64
30	2.09	2.01	1.93	1.89	1.84	1.79	1.74	1.68	1.62
40	2.00	1.92	1.84	1.79	1.74	1.69	1.64	1.58	1.51
60	1.92	1.84	1.75	1.70	1.65	1.59	1.53	1.47	1.39
120	1.83	1.75	1.66	1.61	1.55	1.50	1.43	1.35	1.25
∞	1.75	1.67	1.57	1.52	1.46	1.39	1.32	1.22	1.00

Practical statistics for the health sciences

Table 6 Chi-square distribution

For a particular number of degrees of freedom each entry represents the critical value of χ^2 corresponding to a specified upper tail area α.

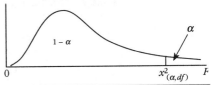

Degrees of freedom	Upper tail areas									
	.995	.99	.975	.95	.90	.10	.05	.025	.01	.005
1	0.000	0.000	0.001	0.004	0.016	2.706	3.841	5.024	6.635	7.879
2	0.010	0.020	0.051	0.103	0.211	4.605	5.991	7.378	9.210	10.597
3	0.072	0.115	0.216	0.352	0.584	6.251	7.815	9.348	11.345	12.838
4	0.207	0.297	0.484	0.711	1.064	7.779	9.488	11.143	13.277	14.860
5	0.412	0.554	0.831	1.145	1.610	9.236	11.071	12.833	15.086	16.750
6	0.676	0.872	1.237	1.635	2.204	10.645	12.592	14.449	16.812	18.548
7	0.989	1.239	1.690	2.167	2.833	12.017	14.067	16.013	18.475	20.278
8	1.344	1.646	2.180	2.733	3.490	13.362	15.507	17.535	20.090	21.955
9	1.735	2.088	2.700	3.325	4.168	14.684	16.919	19.023	21.666	23.589
10	2.156	2.558	3.247	3.940	4.865	15.987	18.307	20.483	23.209	25.188
11	2.603	3.053	3.816	4.575	5.578	17.275	19.675	21.920	24.725	26.757
12	3.074	3.571	4.404	5.226	6.304	18.549	21.026	23.337	26.217	28.299
13	3.565	4.107	5.009	5.892	7.042	19.812	22.362	24.736	27.688	29.819
14	4.075	4.660	5.629	6.571	7.790	21.064	23.685	26.119	29.141	31.319
15	4.601	5.229	6.262	7.261	8.547	22.307	24.996	27.488	30.578	32.801
16	5.142	5.812	6.908	7.962	9.312	23.542	26.296	28.845	32.000	34.267
17	5.697	6.408	7.564	8.672	10.085	24.769	27.587	30.191	33.409	35.718
18	6.265	7.015	8.231	9.390	10.865	25.989	28.869	31.526	34.805	37.156
19	6.844	7.633	8.907	10.117	11.651	27.204	30.144	32.852	36.191	38.582
20	7.434	8.260	9.591	10.851	12.443	28.412	31.410	34.170	37.566	39.997
21	8.034	8.897	10.283	11.591	13.240	29.615	32.671	35.479	38.932	41.401
22	8.643	9.542	10.982	12.338	14.042	30.813	33.924	36.781	40.289	42.796
23	9.260	10.196	11.689	13.091	14.848	32.007	35.172	38.076	41.638	44.181
24	9.886	10.856	12.401	13.848	15.659	33.196	36.415	39.364	42.980	45.559
25	10.520	11.524	13.120	14.611	16.473	34.382	37.652	40.646	44.314	46.928
26	11.160	12.198	13.844	15.379	17.292	35.563	38.885	41.923	45.642	48.290
27	11.808	12.879	14.573	16.151	18.114	36.741	40.113	43.194	46.963	49.645
28	12.461	13.565	15.308	16.928	18.939	37.916	41.337	44.461	48.278	50.993
29	13.121	14.257	16.047	17.708	19.768	39.087	42.557	45.722	49.588	52.336
30	13.787	14.954	16.791	18.493	20.599	40.256	43.773	46.979	50.892	53.672
40	20.707	22.164	24.433	26.509	29.051	51.805	55.758	59.342	63.691	66.766
50	27.991	29.707	32.357	34.764	37.689	63.167	67.505	71.420	76.154	79.490
60	35.534	37.485	40.482	43.188	46.459	74.397	79.082	83.298	88.379	91.952

Table 7 Lower and upper critical values for Wilcoxon signed-rank test

| | One-tailed: $\alpha = .05$ | | $\alpha = .025$ | | $\alpha = .01$ | | $\alpha = .005$ | |
| | Two-tailed: $\alpha = .10$ | | $\alpha = .050$ | | $\alpha = .02$ | | $\alpha = .010$ | |
n	W_L	W_U	W_L	W_U	W_L	W_U	W_L	W_U
5	0	15	-	-	-	-	-	-
6	2	19	0	21	-	-	-	-
7	3	25	2	26	0	28	-	-
8	5	31	3	33	1	35	0	36
9	8	37	5	40	3	42	1	44
10	10	45	8	47	5	50	3	52
11	13	53	10	56	7	59	5	61
12	17	61	13	65	10	68	7	71
13	21	70	17	75	12	79	10	81
14	25	80	21	84	16	89	13	92
15	30	90	25	95	19	101	16	104
16	35	101	29	107	23	113	19	117
17	41	112	34	119	27	126	23	130
18	47	124	40	131	32	139	27	144
19	53	137	46	144	37	153	32	158
20	60	150	52	158	43	167	37	173

Source Adapted from Wilcoxon, F & Wilcox, R A 1964, *Some Rapid Approximate Statistical Procedures,* American Cyanamid Company, New York, by permission of the American Cyanamid Company

Practical statistics for the health sciences

Table 8 Critical values for Mann–Whitney test (5% two-tailed)

n_2 \ n_1	3		4		5		6		7		8		9		10	
	M_l	M_r	M_l	M_r	M_l	M_r	M_l	M_r	M_l	M_r	M_l	M_r	M_l	M_r	M_l	M_r
3	–	–														
4	6	18	11	25												
5	6	21	12	28	18	37										
6	7	23	12	32	19	41	26	52								
7	7	26	13	35	20	45	28	56	37	68						
8	8	28	14	38	21	49	29	61	39	73	49	87				
9	8	31	15	41	22	53	31	65	41	78	51	93	63	108		
10	9	33	16	44	24	56	32	70	43	83	54	98	66	114	79	131

Source Weiss, N A & Hassett, H J 1989, *Introductory Statistics,* 2nd edn, Addison-Wesley Publishing Co Inc, Reading, Massachusetts

Table 9 Critical values for Mann–Whitney test (10% two-tailed)

n_2 \ n_1	3		4		5		6		7		8		9		10	
	M_l	M_r	M_l	M_r	M_l	M_r	M_l	M_r	M_l	M_r	M_l	M_r	M_l	M_r	M_l	M_r
3	6	15														
4	7	17	12	24												
5	7	20	13	27	19	36										
6	8	22	14	30	20	40	28	50								
7	9	24	15	33	22	43	30	54	39	66						
8	9	27	16	36	24	46	32	58	41	71	52	84				
9	10	29	17	39	25	50	33	63	43	76	54	90	66	105		
10	11	31	18	42	26	54	35	67	46	80	57	95	69	111	83	127

Source Weiss, N A & Hassett, H J 1989, *Introductory Statistics,* 2nd edn, Addison-Wesley Publishing Co Inc, Reading, Massachusetts

Table 10 Critical values for Pearson's correlation coefficient r

	Level of significance for one-tailed test			
	.05	.025	.01	.005
df = $n - 2$	Level of significance for two-tailed test			
	.10	.05	.02	.010
1	.998	.997	.999	.999
2	.900	.950	.980	.990
3	.805	.878	.934	.959
4	.729	.811	.882	.917
5	.669	.754	.833	.874
6	.622	.707	.789	.834
7	.582	.666	.750	.798
8	.549	.632	.716	.765
9	.521	.602	.685	.735
10	.497	.576	.658	.708
11	.476	.553	.634	.684
12	.458	.532	.612	.661
13	.441	.514	.592	.641
14	.426	.497	.574	.623
15	.412	.482	.558	.606
16	.400	.468	.542	.590
17	.389	.456	.528	.575
18	.378	.444	.516	.561
19	.369	.433	.503	.549
20	.360	.423	.492	.537
21	.352	.413	.482	.526
22	.344	.404	.472	.515
23	.337	.396	.462	.505
24	.330	.388	.453	.496
25	.323	.381	.445	.487
26	.317	.374	.437	.479
27	.311	.367	.430	.471
28	.306	.361	.423	.463
29	.301	.355	.416	.456
30	.296	.349	.409	.449
40	.257	.304	.358	.393
50	.231	.273	.322	.354
60	.211	.250	.295	.325
70	.195	.232	.274	.302
80	.183	.217	.256	.283
90	.173	.205	.242	.267
100	.164	.195	.230	.254

Practical statistics for the health sciences

Table 11 Critical values for Spearman's rank correlation coefficient r_s

n	$\alpha = 0.10$ $\alpha = 0.05$	$\alpha = 0.050$ $\alpha = 0.025$	$\alpha = 0.02$ $\alpha = 0.01$	$\alpha = 0.010$ $\alpha = 0.005$	←One-tailed ←Two-tailed
5	.900				
6	.829	.886	.943		
7	.714	.786	.893		
8	.643	.738	.833	.881	
9	.600	.683	.783	.833	
10	.564	.648	.745	.794	
11	.523	.623	.736	.818	
12	.497	.591	.703	.780	
13	.475	.566	.673	.745	
14	.457	.545	.646	.716	
15	.441	.525	.623	.689	
16	.425	.507	.601	.666	
17	.412	.490	.582	.645	
18	.399	.476	.564	.625	
19	.388	.462	.549	.608	
20	.377	.450	.534	.591	
21	.368	.438	.521	.576	
22	.359	.428	.508	.562	
23	.351	.418	.496	.549	
24	.343	.409	.485	.537	
25	.336	.400	.475	.526	
26	.329	.392	.465	.515	
27	.323	.385	.456	.505	
28	.317	.377	.448	.496	
29	.311	.370	.440	.487	
30	.305	.364	.432	.478	

Solutions

Chapter 1

1a familes in that city N = 1000
 c statistic: 22, parameter: 430

 b 50 families in his area
 d statistic: 0.72, parameter: 0.87

2a 550 patients currently in hospital
 c 45 min: sample mean

 b average admission time
 d no, sampling variability, yes

Chapter 2

1a The data is categorical
 c region 5 and combined regions 6,7,8
 e 1000%

 b region 3
 d region 3

2a ≈ 390 L/min
 c no

 b ≈ 75 – 130 L/min

3a 3%
 c

 b 67

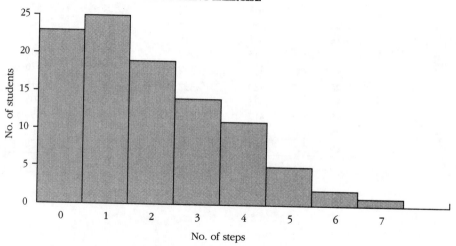

4 0.08, 2.65, 5.67, 44.07, 1.27, 6.23, 2.35, 6.60, 31.08

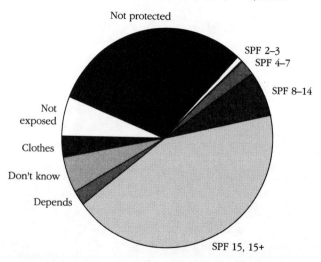

5

Time unemployed (in months)	Number of people
$X < 3$	1379
$3 \leq X < 6$	1800
$6 \leq X < 9$	1513
$9 \leq X < 12$	1220
$12 \leq X$	2647

6

```
Collingwood  |    | Essendon
      0 0 3  | 17 | 2
        8 8  | 17 | 5 8 8 9
  0 3 3 3 4  | 18 | 1 3 3
    5 5 9 9  | 18 | 5 6 8 8 9
  1 2 3 3 4  | 19 | 0 1 2 3
             | 19 | 8 8
          3  | 20 |
             | 20 | 6
```

7

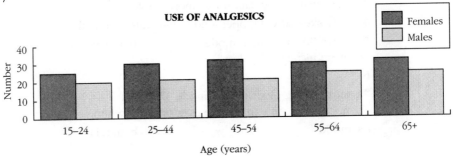

8

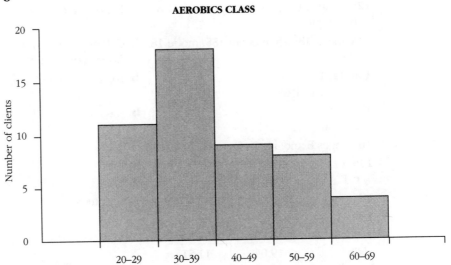

9a

Age	No. of accidents	Relative frequency	Cumulative frequency
5	2	0.019	2
6	10	0.093	12
7	5	0.047	17
8	4	0.037	21
9	5	0.047	26
10	8	0.075	34
11	8	0.075	42
12	14	0.131	56
13	12	0.112	68
14	12	0.112	80
15	16	0.150	96
16	11	0.103	107

c 11.8 years   **d** 32%   **e** 14 years

Chapter 3

1a 14   **b** 2.8

2a μ **b** x bar

3 sensitive to every data point, more stable

4 badly skewed data, open-ended intervals, nominal data

5a mean 3.6, median 4, mode 4   **b** mean changes to 4.3
  c mean increases by 2

6 5

7a mean 37.62, median 37.9, mode 37.9, 38.1
  b no, interest only in change over time   **c** when central point is desired

8a mode   **b** median
  c mean   **d** median

11a 15.44   **b** 14
  c no mode

12a mean 2.607; median 2.4; mode 1.8, 2.1, 2.7; best mean
  b boxplot

13a mean 185.15, median 185, mode 183   **b** Collingwood: Q1 178.5, Q3 191.75
  Essendon: Q1 179.5, Q3 190.75

14a 12, 162 1296   **b** 10, 4480, 40 000
  c 7, 3200, 19 600

15a 648   **b** 4800
  c 2800

16 ranges 8 and 11, St. Devs. 4.178 and 3.317

17a F   **b** T
  c F   **d** T

18 room 1 because of much smaller variation in times

19

	Mean	St. Dev.
Male	19.04	11.51
Female	16.20	10.73

Practical statistics for the health sciences

Chapter 4

1a dependent   **b** independent
 c dependent   **d** independent

4a A = {2,4,6}, B = {4,5,6}, C = {1,2}, D = {3}
 b (i) 1/2   **(ii)** 2/3
   (iii) 1/3   **(iv)** 0
   (v) 1/3

5 Venn diagram
 a 0.1   **b** 0.2
 c 0.1   **d** 0.4
 e 0.55

6a 0.15   **b** 0.95
 c 0.9375

8a 1/10   **b** 1/12
 c 11/60

9 0.2, total probability = 1

10a 0.5   **b** 0.4
  c 0.8   **d** 0.8
  e 1

11a 60/150   **b** 85/150
  c 40/50   **d** 40/85
  e 105/150   **f** no, no

12a 0.17   **b** 0.29, 0.04
  d 0.22   **e** 0.13

Chapter 5

1 0.88

2 0.00024

3 $12.67

4 $5000

5 $88 000

6 $1.78, assuming $3 and $5 represent winnings, otherwise $1.23

7 yes

8 0.74

9 mean 1, variance 1

10 2364.86

11 3.04

12a 0.2757   **b** 0.7439

13a 0.1975   **b** 0.79

14a 0.12386   **b** 0.1738

15a 0.7072   **b** 0.4613
  c 0.1483

16a 0.7196   **b** 0.0781
  c 0.5256   **d** 0.4744

17 0.1240

18a 0.0100	**b** 0.6996
19 0.1916	
20a 0.0102	**b** 0.0870
c 0.6630	
21a 0.1008	**b** 0.4232
c 0.8008	
22a 0.1429	**b** 0.1353
23a 0.0620	**b** 0.4016
24a 0.3233	**b** 0.1353

Chapter 6

1a 0.9236	**b** 0.8133
c 0.2424	**d** 0.0823
e 0.0250	**f** 0.6435
2a 0.35	**b** −1.21
c 2.14	**d** 1.96
3a −1.72	**b** 0.54
c 1.28	
4a 0.9850	**b** 0.0918
c 0.3371	
5a 19.77%	**b** 59.67%
c 1.22%	
6a 0.0548	**b** 0.4514
c 23	**d** 189.95mL
7a 0.0571	**b** 99.11%
c 0.3974	**d** 8.29 am
8a 63.9	**b** 87
c 77.1	
9 75	
10a 8.95	**b** 264.25
c 28	**d** 12.5
11a 4.01%	**b** 94.79%
c 95.44%	**d** 13.36%
e 54.68%	
12 122	
13 6.24 years	
14a 0.8005	**b** 0.7803
15a 0.7925	**b** 0.0352
c 0.0117	
16a 0.8643	**b** 0.2978
c 0.0796	
17a 0.0668	**b** 0.0668
18a 0.9966	**b** 0.123
c 50%	
19a 0.0838	**b** 0.1635
20a 0.0778	**b** 0.017
c 0.6811	

Practical statistics for the health sciences

Chapter 7

1 0.24

2a 0.785 **b** 61.6%

3b 0.634 **c** 0.506, r has decreased
 d 25.6%

4a false **b** true
 c false **d** false

5a 0.857 **b** 0.91

6a 0.846 **b** Exp A 0.697 Exp B 0.750

7b Pearson's r 0.644, Spearman's rho 0.494

8 0.884

9 0.86

10 $r = -0.929$

Chapter 8

1b $Y = -0.02 + 0.316X$ **c** $X = 6.53 - 1.11Y$
 e 3.772

2b contacts = 126 − 1.43 anxiety, negative since contacts decrease as anxiety increases
 c no anxiety expect 126 contacts, contacts decrease by 1.43 for each unit increase in anxiety score
 d 71.66 **e** 47.7%

3a profit = 11.7 − 10.8 Cost **b** 195.3, but this may not be reliable
 c model not reliable, p-values high

4a $Y = 1.76 - 0.168X$ **b** no sound time to respond 1.76, meaningless since patient cannot respond to what they don't hear, response time decreases by 0.168 for each unit increase in sound intensity
  d 0.1968

c 86.3%
 e −0.256 out of range of model

5a $Y = 10.2X + 5$ **b** $Y = 55X$
 c $Y = 27 - 2X$ **d** $Y = 4$

6a Theory = 22.5 + 0.755 Prac **b** 49.4%
 c 11.51 **d** 60.25

7a strong positive linear relationship

8a p-value 0, r-sq 78.1, s 1.388, model is statistically valid and reasonably reliable but s fairly large for this data set
 b for each 1 mm increase in radius, the ulcer will take about one extra week to heal
 c the regression constant is meaningless, as there would be no ulcer
 d no, 15 is well out of the range of the independent variable

Chapter 9

1 statistics are measurements made on samples, whereas parameters are measurements made on populations

2a true **b** false
 c true

3 b

4 a

6 *t*-distribution with 3 degrees of freedom

7 mean 100, variance 0.16

8 mean 50, St. Dev. 2.5

9a 0.3085   **b** 10

  c 0.1587   **d** 2.93 min

10 0.3446

11 0.0475

12 0.2389

13a 0.3161   **b** 1

  c the first probability is for a single commercial, whereas the second probability is for the average cost of a sample of 36 commercials

14 16

15 100

16 a point estimate for a parameter is a single value estimate, whereas an interval estimate provides a range of values within which it is believed the parameter lies

18 b

19 b

20a (52.92, 58.68)   **b** (53.38, 58.22)

21a 7.2   **b** (7.12, 7.28)

22a (583.7, 602.3)   **b** yes

  c between 6% and 7% (interpolating from t-tables)

23 (487.88, 498.22)

24 sample c largest sample (narrowest interval), sample b smallest (widest interval)

25 97.42%

26 c (narrowest)

27 Sample A 240, Sample B 240, Sample C 241

28a (22.90, 25.10)   **b** 1.10 min

  c 24.97

29a (45.87, 49.12)   **b** (40.37, 54.63)

  c 265

30a (8.05, 11.35)   **b** (8.19, 11.21)

  c 36   **d** 94

31 16

32 87

33 196

34 mean 24, St. Dev. 0.3

35a 0.2643   **b** 0.3753

36 0.00012

37 (40.65, 90.75)

38 (4.45, 5.15)

Chapter 10

1a false   **b** true

3a true

4 d

5 a

6 d

7 b (or perhaps d)

8a ± 1.96 **b** -1.645

9a $H_0: \mu = 85$ **b** $H_1: \mu < 85$
   c $Z = -1.29$ **d** reject if $Z < -1.645$
   e true population mean probably not less than 85

10 p = 0.0073, results support claim

11 reject H_0 ($Z = -2.48$)

12 yes ($Z = -2.54$)

13 fail to reject H_0 ($Z = -1.18$)

14 average exceeds 7 days ($p = 0.0044$)

15 small sample, population normal, σ unknown

16a 23   **b** 9
   c 18   **d** 3

17 accept H_0 $t = 1.414$

18 yes (t = 2.88)

19 accept H_0, $t = 2.18$

20 students on average sleep less than 8 hours ($t = -5.16$)

21a $H_0: \mu \geq 15$, $H_1: \mu < 15$ **b** $H_0: \mu \leq 0.008$, $H_1: \mu > 0.008$
   c $H_0: \mu = 16$
      $H_1: \mu \neq 16$

22 (0.408, 0.502)

23 (0.342, 0.475)

24a (0.258, 0.308)   **b** (0.078, 0.144)

25a 246   **b** 385

26 2305

27 fewer than 60% favour increase in tax ($z = -2.19$)

28 less than 70% prefer bottles ($z = 3.06$)

29 $\alpha \leq 0.011$

Chapter 11

1 yes ($p = 0.0037$, $t = 3.67$)

2a $H_1: \mu_1 \neq \mu_2$ **b** $H_0: \mu_1 = \mu_2$
   c Pill does not effect blood pressure ($t = 1.52$)

3 children near smelter have higher lead levels ($p = 0.0019$, $t = 3.81$)

4 not conclusive that these graduates get higher pay ($p = 0.18$, $t = 0.98$)

5a $H_1: \mu_1 > 78$ **b** $H_0: \mu_1 = 78$
   c School mean higher than area mean ($z = 2.62$)

6 advertising does increase sales ($t = 4.10$)

7 depression does interfere with sleep ($t = -2.83$)

8 Reject H_0 $Z = 4.22$, $p = 0$

10 data Op B is not normal

11 no significant difference in fuel economy ($p = 0.37$, $t = 0.34$)

12 the professional unit scored higher on the audit ($t = 5.78$, $p = 0$)

Chapter 12

1 no, p = 0.0310

2 median is not \$85000 ($p = 0.08145$)

3 accept H_0 ($p = 0.071$)

4 reject H_0 ($p = 0.012$)

5 accept H_0 ($p = 0.3437$)

6 conclude that median scores are not equal ($p = 0.0275$)

7 difference in satisfaction is not significant at 0.01 level ($p = 0.1150$)

8 yes (p = 0.0171)

9 p-value for sign test = 0.1719 but for Wilcoxon is 0.063 still accept H_0

10 weight difference not significantly less than 4.5 kg ($p = 0.166$)

11 Mann-Whitney, there is a difference A appears to last longer than B

12 same days, use Wilcoxon reject H_0

13 Mann-Whitney, no ($p = 0.1336$)

14 no, $p = 0.1229$

Chapter 13

1 Distribution is not even throughout the year, $\chi^2 = 40$

2a row totals 322, 368, 60; column totals 31, 51, 226; $N = 750$

  b yes, $\chi^2 = 31.241$

3a 25   **b** no, $\chi^2 = 2.48$

4 yes, $\chi^2 = 52.702$

5 no, $\chi^2 = 1.886$

6 no, too many prunes not enough apple, $\chi^2 = 10.144$

7 results not uniform, more Cs but fewer Bs and Ds than expected, $\chi^2 = 10$

8 hypertension depends on smoking, $\chi^2 = 14.464$

9 TV viewing independent of gender, $\chi^2 = 5.47$

10 number of children independent of education level of mother, $\chi^2 = 7.464$

11 data does fit binomial $\chi^2 = 3.9257$

12 no, $\chi^2 = 5.778$

13 accept H_0 $\chi^2 = 1.0556$

14 no, $\chi^2 = 7.6132$

Chapter 14

1a 24   **b** 5

  c 9.47   **d** 4.53

2 sums of squares between groups and mean square between groups

3 SS error and MS error

4a

	Mean	St. Dev.
Private	413.2	62.86
Service	395.0	75.96
Convenience	479.0	72.68

b $s_B^2 = 11584$, $s_W^2 = 5076$

c s_B^2 measure variance between groups, s_W^2 measures variance within groups

d independent groups, normal distributions, equality of variances

5a between groups, within groups and Total sums of squares

b independent groups, normal distributions, equality of variances

6 no significant differences in mean sales (p = 0.721)

7 courses appear to be of equal difficulty (p = 0.969)

8 moods not effected by weather (p = 0.017)

9

Source	df	SS	MS	
Factor	3	48	16	F = 8.00
Error	36	72	2	
Total	39	120		

At least one mean is significantly different from at least one other mean

Bibliography

Clegg, F 1982, *Simple Statistics*, Cambridge University Press, Cambridge

Jacobs, H R 1970, *Mathematics: A Human Endeavor*, W H Freeman & Company, San Francisco

Pagano, R 1986, *Understanding Statistics in the Behavioral Sciences*, 2nd edn, West Publishing Company, St Paul, Minnesota

Petocz, P 1990, *Introductory Statistics*, Thomas Nelson Australia, Melbourne

Staudte, R G 1990, *Seeing Through Statistics*, Prentice Hall Australia, Sydney

Stevenson, W J 1985, *Business Statistics: Concepts and Applications*, 2nd edn, Harper & Row, New York

Walpole, R E 1989, *Probability and Statistics for Engineers and Scientists*, 4th edn, Macmillan Publishers, New York

Weiss, N A & Hassett, M J 1989, *Introductory Statistics*, 2nd edn, Addison-Wesley Publishing Co Inc, New York

Index

Practical statistics for the health sciences